Linguistic Encounters
with Language Handicap

Linguistic Encounters with Language Handicap

DAVID CRYSTAL

Basil Blackwell

© David Crystal 1984

First published 1984

Basil Blackwell Publisher Ltd
108 Cowley Road, Oxford OX4 1JF, UK

Basil Blackwell Inc.
432 Park Avenue South, Suite 1505,
New York, NY 10016, USA

British Library Cataloguing in Publication Data

Crystal, David
    Linguistic encounters with language handicap.
    1. Language disorders
    I. Title
    616.85'5   RC423

    ISBN 0-631-13869-2

Library of Congress Cataloging in Publication Data

Crystal, David 1941–
    Linguistic encounters with language handicap.

    Bibliography
    Includes index.
    1. Language disorders.   2. Neurolinguistics.
3. Psycholinguistics.   I. Title.
RC423.C77   1984   616.85'5   84-12480
ISBN 0-631-13869-2

Typeset by Stephen Austin, Hertford England
Printed in Great Britain by The Pitman Press Ltd, Bath

Contents

Preface

If the title hadn't already been used, and if the publishers hadn't shown such good sense, this book might have been called 'Close Encounters of the Third (Linguistic) Kind'. The film title reflects the view that there are three stages of contact between man and extraterrestrial life: the first encounter is the sighting of UFOs; the second is the physical evidence of their presence on earth; and the third is actual contact. I am intrigued by the title, because I see in this sequence of events the reflection of my own history of encounter with language handicap.

My first sighting of a UVO (unidentified verbal object) was quite fortuitous. Not long after the Department of Linguistic Science had been established at Reading University, I was rung up by the Audiology Department of the Royal Berkshire Hospital and invited to a case conference being held to discuss a child whose problems were proving to be especially difficult. At the conference, before seeing the child, I was given a set of case notes which I found myself totally unable to understand: my linguistic background had not prepared me for the mixture of medical, audiological and psychological terminology. I was therefore very relieved when, upon seeing the child, I found myself able to make some observations about the language patterns she was using, which seemed to be of interest to other participants. I have not forgotten the elation and frustration of that conference. On the one hand, here were respectable people professing an interest in my subject, and saying it could be helpful; on the other hand, there was a terminological wall which kept us apart, and which made the nature of the handicap curiously unreal and remote.

The result of this first encounter was some five years of further observation, wandering in and out of classrooms and clinics, in an effort to climb the wall of terminology which surrounds the field of language handicap. The relevant literature proved of little help, as it simply added definition to definition: I still have the 50 or so definitions of *aphasia* which I collected at the time (without realizing that there were several dozen more awaiting collection (see Chapter 1)). The clinical visits were much more worthwhile, as they provided an opportunity to collect lists of symptoms, which could then be classified in various ways. After a while, I felt sufficiently confident to try to write something coherent about the relationship between linguistics and language handicap: and this first, distant encounter was published as a paper, 'The case of linguistics: a prognosis', in the *British Journal of Disorders of Communication* in 1972.

The next step was the need to provide physical evidence of these encounters, in the form of a permanent, succinct record of the observed symptoms, which could be used as a basis of comparison. It took a further five years to devise and test the first of the procedures which I felt was needed in order to make progress in assessment and diagnosis. This procedure, focusing on grammatical handicap, was duly published in 1976 (Crystal, Fletcher and Garman). In its preparation, we systematically examined many samples of child and adult language use, and began to develop a clinical sense of what abnormal linguistic patterning comprised. The verbal objects were now becoming more clearly identifiable. This was a close encounter of the second kind.

During this period, we were constantly under pressure to make recommendations concerning remediation. We felt unable to say anything systematic, given the limited research, though a few sporadic, halting suggestions were incorporated in the 1976 work. However, as a result of the contacts we had made with teachers and therapists (referred to as T in this book), especially through in-service courses in clinical linguistic techniques, it proved increasingly possible to develop hypotheses about intervention with patients and pupils (P in this book). The third kind of linguistic encounter, accordingly, came with the systematic investigation of remedial techniques and materials: the linguistic analyses finally made contact with the people they were intended to serve.

I am careful to say that it was the analyses which made contact, and not the linguist, in my case. I am not one of those linguists who wishes to manage as well as analyse P, for two reasons. First, I have no training in management, nor do I feel instinctively that I would be any good at it (an instinct for which there is some evidence, incidentally, as P and I learned to our mutual cost on various occasions when T was absent and I was left in charge!). My métier is analysis, and I am in no doubt that the enormous task of teaching and management (of relatives and parents, as well as of P) is best left for those who find this their vocation. Secondly, it is important, in any enquiry with a research goal, to arrive at an objective statement of the handicap— which includes T's handling of it (see Chapter 5)—and this can be achieved only by someone distancing himself from an interaction. All my current clinical work, therefore, is done at a distance from P: for speech work, I use one-way windows and videotape monitoring, and keep in touch with T by intercom; for reading work, I collaborate with colleagues in teaching in the writing of materials. But though physically distant, I do not feel psychologically distant: when P responds in a teaching situation as the theory predicts he will (see Chapter 5), I do not think I could feel closer.

The present book, then, is an account of my own encounters with language handicap, over a period of some 18 years. It begins with the problem of terminology, and argues that anxiety over terms should be replaced by anxiety over the precise description of symptoms. Chapter 2 outlines the subject of clinical linguistics, which has description as one of its aims. Chapter 3 applies the approach in a general way to the study of two domains of handicap, adult aphasia and specific learning disability. In the course of carrying out this kind of study the importance of a broader perspective emerges, and this is presented in Chapter 4, under the heading of clinical psycholinguistics. Chapter 5 completes the process of encounter by interpreting the general principles of the subject in relation to specific tasks of intervention and materials production. By moving from clinical linguistic theory, through problems of analysis and description, to the principles and practice of remediation, I hope thereby to illustrate the logic of my three stages of encounter, which act as more than a metaphor for this book. Chapter 6 is different: it looks at the future of clinical linguistic studies, and in considering the implications of longitudinal studies of language handicap, arrives at a far-reaching and potentially disturbing conclusion.

Some readers with a good medium-term memory span may recognize parts of this book. Most of Chapter 1 was originally published as a paper in the *British Journal of Disorders of Communication* (1982), and I have retained the title for the chapter. Parts of Chapters 2 and 3 have been given as papers to various conferences in recent years. The section on aphasia in Chapter 3 overlaps with my contribution to *Aphasia* (ed. M. Coltheart *et al.*, to be published by Butterworths in 1985); the section on specific learning disability in the same chapter was originally a contribution to a conference organized by the Berkshire and Oxfordshire Dyslexia Associations in 1983. Chapter 4 is based on a paper given to the XIX International Congress of Logopedics and Phoniatrics, held in Edinburgh in 1983, and published in *Phonetica* (1983). The first section of Chapter 5 develops a conference paper given to a symposium on Research Trends in the Study of Child Language Disability, held at the University of Wisconsin in 1981. All of the material has been extensively revised and reorganized for the present book, and has been supplemented by a great deal of fresh writing, so that the balance of old and new is about even.

The slogan advertising the film *Close Encounters* was: 'We are not alone.' Here, too, life reflects art. It will be evident from the above that without the cooperation of several people, my close encounters would have remained only of the first kind. I am particularly indebted to my co-authors, Paul Fletcher, Michael Garman and John Foster, whose contributions will be evident from the references; to Rita Twiston-Davies, who participated in the terminology project referred to in Chapter 1; and to all those who have been involved in the assessment clinic at Reading University, during the period which led to the writing of this book—in particular, Hilary Crystal, Margaret Davison, Pat Gaffey, Susan Edwards, Carolyn Letts, Chris McConnell, Dr Patricia Scanlon and Marion Trim. The Leverhulme Trust generously provided a grant to enable me to purchase some of the videotapes required. The support of the Medical Research Council is also gratefully acknowledged, in the form of a research grant to enable the detailed analysis of my assessment clinic data to be carried out, the findings of which will be published separately in due course.

David Crystal
March 1984

1

Terms, time and teeth

An evil spirit seems to preside over all branches of clinical language studies. No-one can escape his influence. He sets profession against profession, clinician against clinician, researcher against researcher. He tempts all to follow him, in the name of clarity and precision, but all who do find only obscurity and quicksand. His name is Terminology and his exorcism is the main aim of this chapter.

Anxiety over terminology has been a part of clinical consciousness for generations. In 1917, Elsie Fogerty, one of the founders of British speech therapy, opened a speech clinic at the Westminster Hospital. In Cole's biography of 'Fogie' (1967: p.68), a comment is made of her at the time:

> Disorders of speech had opened up a new field of research, and the early pioneers . . . had perforce to invent their own terminology; unfortunately these pioneers did not always consult each other, so that the classification and terminology might be described as 'confusion worse confounded'.

Moving on 60 years or so, one of the first books to appear in the 1980s on the subject of speech therapy (Byers Brown 1981) contains a discussion of the scope of the profession, after which the following comment is made (p.79):

> There is now a fair degree of consensus among speech therapists as to the conditions requiring treatment.

Unfortunately this consensus does not extend to the terms that should be used to depict the conditions. The need for a clear and comprehensive terminology is everywhere expressed but not yet satisfied.

The focus on terminology can be seen in the repeated attempts to provide glossaries of terms—some, fairly short lists; others, attempts at full-scale dictionaries. A relatively early example is Robbins (1951); a recent example of the same genre is Nicolosi, Harryman and Kresheck (1978). The focus can be seen, less formally, in the correspondence columns of professional journals and newsletters, where terminological disquiet over everything from clinical entities to the name of the profession—especially the latter—has become a routine space-filler. It can be seen in severe form in training courses to do with linguistic handicap, where students may be presented with a range of conflicting and overlapping terms, not all of which are easily relatable to their ongoing clinical experience (a particular motivation for Byers Brown's discussion). And it can be seen, most disturbingly, in the disunity apparent in case-notes and case-conferences between professionals of different disciplines, or of different persuasions within a discipline, when a conflict over terms can symbolize deep-rooted differences of opinion concerning matters of diagnosis or treatment. All modalities of communication have been affected: the problem is just as noticeable in hearing as in speech, in relation to both reading and writing (as the long-standing debate over the application of such terms as *dyslexia* and *specific learning disability* illustrates (see further, Chapter 3)), and increasingly in relation to the burgeoning industry of alternative communication systems (where, for example, the labelling of such systems as *codes, languages,* or whatever, continues to generate much emotion). The problem of terminology is by no means restricted to the British setting, but has attracted the recent interest of groups in America, Australia and South Africa. Nor is it a problem restricted to English, as a glance at almost any continental conference proceedings within the field of logopaedics or phoniatrics will indicate (e.g. Perello 1977).

So we have a problem, as the astronauts say—which, after

several decades of study, does not seem to be resolving. Indeed, the popular impression is that it is getting worse. What, then, can be done?

The general situation

Let us first put the problem in perspective. The field of linguistic handicap is by no means the first to encounter the terminological devil. Confused terminology affects all domains of thinking, and all languages. The point has now been officially recognized, by the setting-up of several international bodies whose prime concern is to keep in touch with terminological developments in different fields and countries, and provide networks for coordination. For example, there is the International Information Centre for Terminology (Infoterm), set up by UNESCO and Austria. The EEC employs several full-time terminologists in its Translation and Terminology Section. Most international subject-orientated bodies (such as the World Health Organization, or the World Meteorological Organization) collaborate with the International Organization for Standardization (ISO). And while these organizations are mainly concerned with terminological issues to do with the pure and applied physical sciences, medicine and mental health have also attracted a great deal of attention, and it is here that some concern over the terminology of linguistic handicap has been shown (see Sager and Johnson 1978, Krommer-Benz 1977, Tymchuk 1973, World Health Organization 1974).

What sort of findings have emerged from the research carried on by these bodies? An important early discovery was that the word 'terminology' is itself in need of definition! It has three main senses. Its most obvious sense is 'the system of terms belonging to a specialized subject'. In this sense, a terminologist would study what terms there are, how they relate to each other, how they are formed, how they are defined, and so on. Note that this definition makes no reference to 'concepts', 'knowledge structure', or the like. For example, in chemistry there is a pair of terms, *molality* and *molarity*. The latter term has nothing to do with your ability to bite. One dictionary defines it as 'the number of moles of solute per litre of solution'. The former term is defined as 'the number of moles of solute per litre of solvent'. Now, I cite these definitions because, having done so, I imagine most readers of this chapter are none the wiser. Yet the definitions will have made a certain amount of sense, being evidently concerned with quantities. Further reference to the dictionary would show that mole is here not an insectivorous mammal, nor a secret agent, but a short form referring to the molecular weight of a substance, expressed in grams; *molal* is an adjective derived from *mole; solute* is a substance which has been dissolved in a given solution; and so on. After all this, I think it would be possible to make sense of the definitions—but most readers would still be none the wiser. I now know exactly what molarity and molality mean, and could handle them with ease on *Call My Bluff*, but if I was taken into a chemistry laboratory, I would not be able to recognize these two processes when they occur, or tell the difference between them, or know how to calculate a mole, or distinguish a solution from a solvent. In short, I have no sense of the knowledge structure which this language represents. But, as a terminologist, I could still study the differences between these definitions, show how *molal* has become *molality*, whereas *mole* has become *molarity*, and so on. I could look the words up in various dictionaries, to see whether they all define them in the same way—or I could ask various chemists or look in various textbooks (which is of course what the dictionary-writers did in the first place). Most important of all, I could check to see whether identical processes of word formation had taken place between different languages. It would be silly if *molarity* did not correspond to *molarité* in French; it would be nice if the neat parallelism between *molarity* and *molality* could be found in other languages. There are obviously many such issues which can interest me as a terminologist of chemistry—even though I would make a rotten chemist!

The second sense of *terminology* is quite different in this respect. Here, we are referring to the concepts as well as the terms of a special field. A terminologist, in this sense, asks some rather different questions. He is more concerned with evaluative matters. Is such-and-such a term needed? Is it an adequate reference to the phenomenon it was devised to describe? Is it relevant, in modern times? Is it an important term, representing a concept central to the identity of the subject? To go back to my example of *molarity* and *molality*. Is this an up-to-date distinction? Is it universally used amongst chemists? Does it represent a particular school of thought or point of view? Would one be likely to find the distinction in a first-year school text on the subject, or is it a degree-level notion? Such questions—of whether a subject has too many, or too few, or the right kind of terms—are obviously of great importance, but because they cannot be answered without a genuine understanding of the subject, they are very different in kind from those subsumed under my first sense of *terminology*.

The third sense of *terminology* raises a set of more general theoretical or methodological issues. Here we are concerned with the extent to which universal strategies for handling specialized vocabulary can be established—regardless of language or subject-matter. Is there anything in common between the way in which chemistry, physics, medicine, and so on develop their terminologies? Are there processes common to all languages—in their use of prefixes, Greek roots, or whatever? Are there universally applicable methods for presenting the information—for example, how to lay out a classified vocabulary, how to make cross-references, or how best to use computer storage facilities (a *sine qua non* of terminological research these days). How might one formally evaluate the properties of different terminological systems? Do different systems have different goals? Are there different popular or specialist attitudes to terminology which need to be taken into account?

I think there are certain important guidelines we can draw from this general orientation. Firstly, we are not alone. Our terminological responsibility is not a parochial one, but to the larger English-speaking community in the first instance, and then beyond that, to the world as a whole. All of us have terms which are dear to us, either because we grew up with them, or invented them, or remember the personality of those who used them. But terms, and the concepts they represent, transcend their creators— or at least, they should. They must be judged according to criteria which, as far as possible, should be universally applicable; in other words, as far as linguistic handicap is concerned, applicable to all languages, and objectively demonstrable as relating to specific sets of medical or behavioural factors. It is not difficult to find terms in this field which break both of these criteria.

Secondly, the search for universal terminological status must be recognized as a long-term goal. It is not something which a field can sort out within a few years, or even a generation. The early terminology of many subjects was just as personal, situationally restricted, anecdotal and tentative as that often encountered in the literature on linguistic handicap. In some cases, it has taken several hundred years to achieve a terminology which is universally intelligible and acceptable. In the field of language pathology, progress had to wait for the development of appropriately sophisticated techniques of investigation, both medical and behavioural. Some people date the beginning of the scientific era of study of this field as 1861, when Paul-Pierre Broca presented his first findings. Personally, I prefer 1877, when Thomas Edison invented the phonograph—or possibly 1935, when the magnetic tape recorder was devised. But whatever one thinks, we are still dealing with a period which is best counted in tens of years rather than hundreds. Compare the situation in medicine. Just over 200 years ago, let it be recalled, Newton thought that nerves were filled with aether, and Dr. Johnson's definition of *spleen* was 'one of the viscera ... the seat of anger, melancholy, and mirth'. With the advent of electronic instrumentation, long-term goals no longer seem as long-term as they used to—but even so, I should be surprised to see a reasonable consolidation of our linguistic terminology before the turn of the century.

Thirdly, a clear distinction needs to be borne in mind between the descriptive phase of terminological enquiry and any prescriptive phase which might follow. What has to be guarded against is premature and uncontrolled prescriptivism. 'Prescriptivism', in this context, refers to the concern for terminological standardization—that practitioners should adopt a single set of terms for use throughout their discipline. This is the point made most insistently by speech therapists, in their critique of the current situation. But two factors need to be remembered. First, concerning control: any demand for total standardization is unreal and stultifying. If everything is standardized, how can there be any

room for creative interpretation? If everything is standardized, how can the field assimilate discoveries—changes in the knowledge structure which the terminology represents? We must avoid the jigsaw puzzle view of terminological development—that there is a theoretical 'sum of knowledge' which will be pieced together, as research findings accumulate, with each new piece having no effect on the identity of the other pieces already in place. The reality is the opposite: more of a rush-hour tube-train view of terminological development, where a new piece of knowledge elbows its way into the existing terminological situation, forcing some terms out, making some give way, permitting a few solid terms to stand, and generally feeling somewhat uncomfortable for a while, until the other terms settle down and accept the situation. A terminological system, in other words, has to be sufficiently flexible to permit the necessary give and take as new ideas come, and old findings become outdated.

The other factor concerns the prematurity of any move towards standardization. Before we can think of standardizing, we must first be sure what the facts are: how many terms exist, referring to a particular state of affairs; whether their definitions are in fact identical; whether they operate at the same stylistic level; and so on. This information does not conveniently exist in a single place: it has to be researched, in a *descriptive* phase of terminological enquiry. Who uses what terms? When, where, and why? Until we can establish the range of terminological vacillation precisely and comprehensively, any standardization policy remains arbitrary. Unfortunately, in the field of linguistic handicap, too little of this basic descriptive spade-work has been done. The history of use of most of the main terms has not been traced in the degree of detail required. The outline history of the term *dyslalia* given in Byers Brown (1981: pp.86-7) is nice, but it lacks the comprehensive citational support which terminological scholarship requires (from, in this case, both American and British usage). The extent of the problem becomes apparent only when we try to provide this citational support in a full and representative manner—as a recent experience of my own illustrates.

A terminological survey?

In the late 1970s, I was asked to initiate a terminology project, on behalf of the British College of Speech Therapists. The aim of the project was to provide some alternative for the College's terminology leaflet, which had been attracting increasing criticism. Given the limitations of time and financial resources, all that could be achieved was a small-scale study, designed to establish the nature of the difficulty. The first aim was to be a descriptive study of a selection of terms, to establish the range of terminological variation which existed. The second aim was to be a series of recommendations, which would provide the basis for a local (British) standardization, in respect of these terms. The third aim was to provide a model of presentation, which would enable the terminological data to be put to general use. The project certainly succeeded in its general intention, to establish the nature of the difficulty. Indeed, it was too successful in this respect, for the difficulties quickly came to dominate the work, and only the first aim was actually achieved. It remains to be seen whether any kind of product can be salvaged from the study. In the meantime, it is extremely instructive to examine the aetiology of the difficulties, and to arrive at an assessment of the present state of affairs.

The first thing to do was to establish a data-base for the project, and this took the form of all the standard textbooks on speech pathology in current use, the main dictionaries, and any journal articles which were known to discuss terminological matters relevant to the terms being studied. In all, about 50 such texts were routinely consulted, representing British, American and European sources, written mainly by speech pathologists, but including the work of others (neurologists, linguists, etc.) with a special interest in the field. Topics studied included articulation, apraxia, aphasia, dysarthria, language delay, deviance, and many more—each, of course, subsuming several other terms. There was no principle governing the selection of terms, apart from our clinical intuitions about the importance of the terms in the field. We studied articulation disorders first, because we felt that this would be a fairly straightforward area. (We were wrong, as will be apparent below. So much for clinical intuitions!) Other terminological areas were added when they came up naturally enough in routine reading; and we stopped the collection of data when enough material had been accumulated to enable us to identify the nature of the problem.

The detailed procedure took the following form. A textbook would be scrutinized for its information about a certain term, and any definition provided would be copied or photocopied onto a card. This sometimes had to be done more than once for a given author: slight differences in definitional form often occur between one end of a book and another, and these differences had to be noted (not to have done so would have been to commit the sin of prescriptive standardization). For example, Martin has the following to say in an important article on the term *apraxia of speech* (1974: p.54):

Apraxia of speech is a faulty programming of movements and sequences of movements for speech ... By definition, it is a disturbance of encoding that is free of impairment of perceptual decoding.

Later on in the same article (p.58), he says:

Apraxia of speech denotes an encoding impairment that is essentially free from impairment of perceptual decoding.

Note the addition of the word *essentially*, and the change from encoding *disturbance* to *impairment*. Are these modifications trivial or full of consequence for our view of the disorder? One can imagine the kind of debate which might ensue. But for our purposes, as descriptive lexicographers, we do not have to take sides: *both* definitions must be given cards, in this first stage of the investigation.

Once all the terminological information had been extracted from our corpus, a synthesis of the information was made, to see where the consensus of opinion for a particular usage lay. Each definition would be analysed for its distinctive semantic characteristics, and these would be transferred to a summary chart. For example, the *apraxia of speech* definition above would have provided the following items:

> faulty programming
> movements/sequences of movements
> encoding
> disturbance (defn.1)/impairment (defn.2)
> perceptual decoding
> free of impairment (defn.1)/essentially free (defn.2)

I shall give a complete illustration of this procedure below, but first I must refer to the main methodological difficulties in trying to make a procedure of this kind work. It sounds as if it is a quite automatic and thoroughly boring procedure. In fact it is neither automatic nor boring. Isolating terms and extracting definitions engages the critical intellect right from the outset.

First, the question of terms. So far, I have assumed something that cannot be assumed at all—that we know when a word is a term. In fact, it is often unclear whether an author intends his use of a word to be taken in a special sense. Sometimes there is 'systematic ambiguity', with a word being used apparently technically on one page, and then in its everyday sense on the next. Sometimes, variation is introduced, apparently for stylistic reasons (cf. *articulation disorder, articulatory disorder, disordered articulation, disorder of articulation,* etc.), but it is premature to assume that such changes are always stylistic. One of the biggest problems facing the lexicographer of linguistic handicap is what to do with the set of terms that characterize the nature of the impairment—such terms as *disorder, defect, disturbed, deficiency, disability, handicap, inability, incorrect, error, difficulty with,* and so on. There are over 50 such designations. Are they terms at all? Several carry definite implications, some to do with degree of severity, some to do with type of professional background (the sociological nuance for *deprivation,* for instance), and several authors make quite specific distinctions between certain of them, e.g. Berry and Eisenson's distinction between a speech *error* and a speech *defect* (1956: p.36). I suspect that this proliferation of 'inadequacy' terms will be very much in the firing line, when the revolution comes.

The problem of what counts as a term, however, pales alongside the problem of what counts as a definition. If you think that definitions should be of the classical Aristotelian form 'An X is a Y which has/does Z', then you are not likely to be satisfied with the literature on linguistic handicap. When a term is introduced, what we are usually given is not so much a definition, more a *characterization* of a phenomenon; sometimes we are given no definition at all, the author proceeding to a classification directly; and sometimes there is neither definition nor classification, but simply an illustration, which may be systematic or anecdotal. In all cases bar the first (clear definition), the author's exposition may continue through several sentences—or even pages. Here is an example of what I mean. First, something which is clearly a definition (note, I do not say that I find the definition clear—that is a matter about which a decision will have to be made, but at a later stage of the enquiry). Hall Powers (1963) gives a full definition of *functional articulation disorder*:

> a functional articulation disorder can be defined as an inability to produce correctly all of the standard speech sounds of the language, an inability for which there is no appreciable structural, physiological, or neurological basis in the speech mechanism or its supporting structures, but which can be accounted for by normal variations in the organism or by environmental or psychological factors.

A good example of a characterization is Morley's account of *developmental articulatory apraxia* in *The Development and Disorders of Speech in Children*. I shall use the text of the third edition (1972: p.274) which is a slightly expanded version of the second edition (p.237). I shall also add in parentheses the places in this account which present the lexicographer with serious methodological problems:

> Developmental articulatory apraxia, or dyspraxia in its less severe form [which sense of *or* is intended here? exclusive or

inclusive?] has been described [by whom? Morley? others? Morley agreeing with others? or will she disagree with others?] as an inability to perform voluntary movements of the muscles involved in articulation although automatic movements of the same muscles are preserved. [Note also the use of the verb *describe* here—equivalent to *defined*?] It may also be described [*may* = permission? general possibility? generalization?] as a defect of articulation which occurs when the movements of the muscles used for speech, that is tongue, lips, palate or cheeks [only these muscles? Jaw, pharynx, etc. purposely excluded?] appear normal for involuntary and spontaneous [synonyms?] movements, such as smiling or licking the lips, [plainly illustrative here, hence excludable] or even for [unclear what definitional status to assign to what follows] the voluntary imitation of movements carried out on request, but the control and direction [both notions essential?] of articulatory movements is inadequate for the complex and rapid [both notions essential?] movements for articulation and the reproduction [sense? = spontaneous? imitation? both?] of the sequences of sounds used in speech.

In this account, we are given a full picture of the kind of thing involved, but it is by no means clear to the lexicographer—or, for that matter, to the research clinician—which aspects of the account Morley would see as obligatory, and which are optional features of any definition of the phenomenon. This is a very common problem in using textbooks as data for lexicographical analysis, but the poor student of the subject, who does not have the clinical experience to provide a context for disambiguation, can often be confused by precisely these indeterminacies, and penalized for them. To illustrate this point, the reader might care to act as an examiner, and mark the following passage taken from a student essay, concerning the term *dysarthria*:

This term implies slow, clumsy articulation arising from dysfunction of the muscles used in speech. Such dysfunction is evident on physical examination. It does not necessarily involve any interference with the comprehension and formulation of words, although in some children with developmental aphasia there may be associated dysarthria.

Previous examiners, to whom I have presented this extract, have taken issue with 'implies' ('Is it or isn't it?', wrote one in the margin), and many object to 'does not necessarily'. No-one gives it very high marks. In fact (as may already have been perceived) the student who wrote this had copied it out, word for word, from Morley (1972: p.160)!

Let us now look in more detail at a full lexical account of a term. (There is no space to present the whole description here, but only the main headings; nor will I give bibliographical details.*)

articulation disorder also known as *disorder of articulation, disordered articulation, articulatory disorder, abnormality of articulation, articulatory defect, defective articulation, defective use of articulation, defect of articulation, articulation error, articulatory error, articulation problem, articulatory-resonatory disorder, articulation syndrome, dyslalia, misarticulation, impaired articulation* . . .

The general characterization of the abnormality makes reference to a wider range of notions, including: *defective, disturbed, incorrect, deviant, imprecise, confused, difficult to correct, resistant to therapy.* Many definitions make reference to some notion of a community standard, such as: *deviates too far from standard/norm, varies too widely from average values, nonstandard, unacceptable, reduced adult system, falls significantly below our proper expectations.* Some definitions make reference to the role of the speaker (e.g. *degree of speaker awareness, inaccurate judgement of his own sounds*); some to the role of the listener (e.g. *noticeability, unintelligible, attracts attention and disturbs communication*); some refer to both; some specifically exclude both.

Definitions generally refer to *speech production*, but optionally

*The full project details, including the textual sources, will be published separately in due course. The definitions below are taken from Van Riper and Irwin (1958), Emerick and Hatten (1974), Morley and Fox (1969), and Milisen (1966).

add references to *placement, timing, direction, pressure, speed, integration, feedback,* and other such notions.

The quantity of articulations involved merits attention in some definitions. Some make a general observation (e.g. the articulations are *restricted, incomplete, reduced, absent*); some are more specific (e.g. *single sounds, particular groups of sounds, consonants rather than vowels, certain consonants*); some refer to frequency, and some to consistency (e.g. *fairly stable, not necessarily consistent, are inconsistent, inconsistent in imitation task, no generalization to all contexts*).

The nature of the linguistic units involved attracts considerable differences of opinion. First, they are said to be *phonetic* units (*speech sounds* is the usual term here). Secondly, they are said to be *phonemes* (authors use such phrases as *specific phonemes, phonemic system, phonemic difficulty, phonemic discrimination* — and one author includes *prosody*). Thirdly, they are said to be *distinctive features* (e.g. *perception of contrasting features, not necessarily all phonetic features in error, little feature generalization*). Fourthly, some definitions give only a general reference to *sound system, repertoire, patterns,* and the like.

Several definitions involve a reference to the higher-order units affected by the disorder, introducing such concepts as *sound/ syllable/ word patterns, affecting/affected by grammar, dependent on syntactic form and prosody,* or *part of total pattern of communicative response*.

The descriptive classification is usually made with reference to the notions of *omission, substitution* and *distortion* of sounds— though some definitions make reference to *addition* and *transposition*. However, even this is not as straightforward as it seems at first sight. Some definitions state omission, without further qualification; some refer specifically to consonant omissions; one refers especially to weakly stressed consonants. What counts as an *omission*, technically, is also not entirely clear. In this literature *omission* does not always mean 'leaving something out'. To take just one example, the child who says *dog* as [do:]—has he left out the [g], or is the [g] somehow represented by the vowel length? Providing a definition of the notion of *omission* to encompass such problems is by no means easy.

Everything so far has related to the question of behavioural definition. However, about half of the definitions make reference to aetiological factors. Some refer to difficulties in *organic production*—anatomical (e.g. reference to *body structure, physical disabilities, orofacial disabilities, structural anomalies*) and neurophysiological (e.g. reference to *motor coordination, neuromuscular integration, fine neural movements, neural deficiencies*). On the other hand, several refer to *organic reception* problems—either general (e.g. *general sensory deprivation, sensory deficits, sensitivity to auditory stimuli*) or specific (e.g. *reduced auditory acuity, auditory discrimination*). Then, quite a number refer primarily to *non-organic* or *functional* factors: developmental (using such phrases as *delay, slow development, retarded, atypical development, fail to master, persist in immature usage*), social (such as *environmental, cultural, parental maladjustment, personal adjustment*) or psychological (such as *mental retardation, faulty learning, emotional, behavioural, intelligence*).

We can see how all these factors come together if we take a selection of the (shorter) definitions used in the literature:

(a) defective production of a specific phoneme (Van Riper and Irwin 1958: p.1);

(b) substitutions, distortions, omissions and transpositions of the sounds of speech (College of Speech Therapists leaflet);

(c) act of producing speech sounds which deviate too far from the standard set by society (Milisen 1966: p.308);

(d) a nonstandard production of one or more speech sounds (Emerick and Hatten 1974: p.131);

(e) the production of sounds used in speech deviates sufficiently from the standards expected as to interfere with communication (Morley and Fox 1969: p.151); and compare the Hall Powers definition quoted on p.11.

I should perhaps stress, at this point, that the term *articulation disorder* is by no means atypical in its lexicographical complexity; there are others which are far worse (*aphasia* being the worst of all). But it is a good example of the nature of the problems facing the enquirer into terminology. Indeed, it illustrates perfectly the primary problem—that before we go very far into the terminological swamp, the terminology issue pales beside a host of theoretical and empirical questions. The above definitions are often ambiguous, overlapping and sometimes contradictory; and they are often inspecific, in the sense that it is not clear whether their *failure* to mention a factor is deliberate policy or fortuitous. Take the following problems, raised by the above classification:

(a) Is articulation disorder an organic or a non-organic condition? Precisely what range of aetiological factors are involved? Is there any clear correlation with severity of condition?

(b) Is it a phonetic or a phonological disorder? The traditional view is that 'sounds' are affected; the more recent view is that 'sound contrasts' are affected. The issue is confused by the frequent use of the term *phoneme* to mean 'speech sound' instead of 'abstract unit', which is the modern sense. Some authors distinguish between terms for phonetic and phonological disorders (*articulation problem* and *articulation disorder*, in one case).

(c) What is the nature of the units within which the distribution of the articulation disability may be defined (e.g. syllable, word . . .)?

(d) Is this a single disorder varying in severity, or are there sub-types? Should severity be defined with reference to the extent that the child system differs from adults, or with reference to the number and type of sounds affected?

(e) Should other phonological notions be brought into the definition—such as phonological processes?

While there are several theoretical issues raised here, it seems plain to me that the primary problem is an empirical one—questions to do with the frequency, consistency and range of the units affected in speech, or the correlation with factors in the medical history. So little is actually known about the facts of the condition that generalization (and hence definition) must be premature. In the whole of the terminology project, I have found very few examples of simple terminological confusion, in fact—that is, with more than one term referring to exactly the same clinical entity. In most cases, when terms change, the entities change too—sometimes subtly, sometimes grossly. And to have one term for a variety of clinical entities is commonplace (e.g.

dyspraxia, delay). In other words, terminological unclarity may exist, but the cause lies not in the terms themselves but in our uncertain grasp of the clinical symptoms to which they refer. There can be no rational terminology without an accurate and comprehensive symptomatology.

The need for comprehensive description

An accurate and comprehensive symptomatology. It is here that the dangers of using clinical or educational tests as part of research procedures are most in evidence. These tests (articulation tests, for example) have an essential routine role, and are used to excellent effect every day. But by their nature they are highly selective, both in terms of the number of features included, and their distribution and context of use. They cannot give a complete account of the nature of a disorder, for that is not their purpose. Hence to use a test in the empirical investigation of a condition at research level is full of dangers, in that researchers will see only what the test lets them see. Because articulation tests generally test only consonants, and not vowels, for example, there is a general view that difficulties with vowels do not enter into the condition I have been discussing. I do not share this view, for I have seen profile descriptions of several Ps (i.e. patients or pupils) whose vowel systems are grossly impaired. Indeed, a safer hypothesis for the investigation of articulation disorders is that there is *usually* something wrong with the vowel system in such cases (vowel length being a source of particular difficulty, with its concomitant effects on stress and rhythm).

We cannot solve the empirical issues by a rigorous programme of testing. The matter is more fundamental, requiring a more comprehensive approach, and it is here that my own main research interests lie, and not in clinical lexicography at all. In looking back over the whole field of linguistic handicap, insofar as I am able, I am struck by one amazing fact: that, to date, there has been no single published account of *all* aspects of a patient's or pupil's disability, in linguistic terms. There have of course been innumerable fragments, of varying degrees of accuracy. But when we consider all the variables—a complete account of the grammatical constructions used, a complete account of the phonology (including intonation, stress, and other prosodic and paralinguistic features; see further, Chapter 2), a complete account of the semantics (from both grammatical and lexical points of view), a complete account of the sociolinguistic interaction between P and others, a complete account of the psycholinguistic factors affecting P's performance—it is evident that we have a long way to go before even an approximation to comprehensiveness is achieved, for even a single sample. I do not doubt that there are such approximations hidden in case records up and down the country, and I have seen some good moves in this direction in the case studies of students. But there is nothing in the scientific literature, which is where it has to be, if genuine progress is to be made. Even more worrying, from the point of view of speech therapy or remedial language teaching, there is no comparably detailed published *longitudinal* account either—that is, an account of the spontaneous or therapeutically managed progress of P over a period of time—which is a prerequisite step in the development of our ideas about the efficacy of therapeutic strategies (see Chapter 6).

The reason for this unhappy state of affairs is not inherent in the stage that language analysis has reached, as a theoretical enterprise. Adequate prosodic analyses of speech have been around for decades, as have grammatical analyses; and while adequate semantic, sociolinguistic and psycholinguistic analyses are still some way off, there is a great deal that can be done using simple measures of vocabulary range and type, and basic pragmatic criteria. I can put this another way: all that is needed is a level of descriptive achievement which is at least *comparable* to that routinely achieved in other branches of applied language work. We might note the descriptive detail obtained in the stylistic analysis of texts, for example (cf. Crystal and Davy 1969); or accounts of linguistic behaviour in foreign language teaching (cf. Crystal and Davy 1975); or the level of thoroughness provided in child language research (e.g. Wells 1980). Or again, if I have students who express an interest in Turkish or Sindhi, I will send them over to the library to read a descriptive outline or handbook of the language. I would dearly like to be able to send one of my language pathology students over to the library also, to obtain a *descriptive* account of a dyspraxic patient, or a stammerer, or a language delayed child—or *anyone!*

This is why, in the early 1970s, I began my research programme, the principles of which were published in Crystal (1972). The long-term aim was to provide a set of descriptive accounts of the various clinical syndromes, to enable precise differential diagnoses to be made, with accurate assessments, and principled bases for remedial intervention. But it proved impossible to proceed to the empirical task directly. There were no methods available to carry out the task. I could not use traditional tests, for the reasons I have already given; and there were no clinical linguistic procedures of sufficient generality (Lee (1966) was available, for example, but that was for children only, whereas I wanted something for adults as well; also, it dealt only with grammar, whereas other levels of analysis had to be covered too). Accordingly, it proved necessary to invent some; and the first of necessity's children was duly published, after several preliminary versions and clinical trials, in 1976 (Crystal, Fletcher and Garman). This was a procedure for grammatical description—an area which we chose to concentrate on first, because at the time that seemed to be where guidelines were most urgently needed. (The procedure was identified by its acronym LARSP, standing for 'Language Assessment, Remediation and Screening Procedure'. This was not the best of acronyms, given the focus on grammar, but the alternative—to have called it a 'Grammatical Assessment'—would undoubtedly have led to the acronym GRARSP, and we did not wish to hear of therapists 'grarsping' their patients!) We were never exclusively concerned with grammar, however, and once LARSP was published, it was possible to develop the other profiles which I hoped would help to plug the methodological gaps. The first of these to appear was the non-segmental phonological profile, which focused on prosody, and which is known as PROP (Prosody Profile); later came the segmental phonological profile known as PROPH (Profile in Phonology); and lastly, two semantic profiles known as PRISM (Profile in Semantics), one for grammatical semantics and one for

lexical semantics. These have been in use in a special assessment
clinic at Reading since 1978. The theoretical background to these
procedures was published in Crystal (1981), and the first full-
scale exposition of these approaches, along with the profile charts,
appeared shortly afterwards (Crystal 1982a). Work on other
aspects of clinical description is in progress.

The concept of *profile* is pivotal in all this. A linguistic profile is
a principled description of just those features of a person's (or
group's) use of language which will enable him or her to be
identified for a specific purpose. In the present context, the
purpose is to enable an accurate assessment of P's disability to be
made, sufficient to provide a basis for remedial intervention. The
aim is to generate hypotheses concerning the nature of the
disability and its remediation, which it is the purpose of subsequent intervention to confirm or disconfirm. There are thus
two main goals: (a) to identify the linguistic level Ps have
achieved, in relation to the level they should be achieving; and (b)
to suggest a remedial path, which will take them from where they
are to where they ought to be. The main difficulty in all this
research—and the main reason why procedures take so long to
come out (five years, on average)—arises out of the opposed
demands of routine clinical or remedial practice and academic
diagnostic research. Ts (therapists and teachers) are currently
faced with a savage and frustrating conflict of criteria. On the one
hand, there is a growing realization of the highly complex and
individual patterns characteristic of language handicap, and of the
gap between methods of traditional training and the findings of
current research. There is a concern to learn as much as possible
about the problems facing individual Ps, in order to provide them
with the best possible teaching, and to safeguard T against
charges of professional ineptitude. On the other hand, the
demands made on T's time, arising out of heavy caseloads/pupil
ratios, lack of secretarial help, and other well-known factors,
preclude the in-depth study which is ideally required as a solid
foundation for remedial work. It was my hope that linguistic
profiles would provide a method of bridging the gap between the
demands of theory and the exigencies of practice. By reducing the
number of descriptive categories on each chart to a certain

minimum, and grading them in certain ways, it was thought possible (a) to give Ts a tool capable of being used routinely, once the concepts involved had been mastered; and (b) to give those interested in clinical or remedial research a tool which was sufficiently sophisticated to enable properly detailed diagnostic statements to be made. In the event, I think the balance obtained is about right: the criticism of LARSP by Ts on the grounds that it is too complex and time-consuming is just about matched by the criticism of academic linguists that it is oversimplified and not sufficiently explanatory!

To be sure, what must be appreciated by Ts is how elementary a descriptive tool a procedure like LARSP is. There is a tendency in some quarters to identify LARSP with 'doing linguistics'—an identification which does no justice to either. The same point applies to the other profiles referred to above. They are little more than systematic frameworks which enable us to describe samples of linguistic handicap in a comprehensive and graded way. They are the simplest of tools, which will enable us to do the job which needs to be done—the precise identification of the linguistic symptoms of the various forms of handicap. LARSP, PROP, PROPH, PRISM and other such procedures are not 'the research': they are the tools we need in order to get any descriptive research done at all. The *real* research has hardly begun. The real research will take the form of the establishment of linguistic and phonetic syndromes, based on aggregates of phonetic, phonological, grammatical, semantic and other criteria. A large number of such syndromes exist within the broad categories of 'language delay' and 'Broca's aphasia', for example. And, when these syndromes come to be demonstrated, they will be given names (see further, Chapter 4). Then, and only then, will the older, broader and thus emptier terms (such as 'delay') fall into desuetude. It will take a long time, but that is to be expected.

How much time it will take depends largely on how many people involve themselves in this kind of research. I can provide a long-term estimate, but only if I am given an indication of how much short-term time outlay we can rely upon. For who is to do all this research? Should it be clinical linguists? Not solely, for their training does not usually allow them to have a first-hand experience of all the variables. If the 'whole patient' (or pupil) is the focus of the enterprise, then a balance must be struck between the linguistic descriptions which provide the initial symptomatology, and the psychological, social, educational and medical descriptions which accompany them. (There is work to be done under these other headings too, such as more refined analyses of cognitive development, but that is another story.) In my view, the research has to be done by the speech therapists and the remedial language teachers—the people whose professional identity, it seems to me, lies precisely in their ability to integrate, interpret and implement these descriptive findings through patient (in both senses) interaction.

'But we have no time.' This is the criticism most commonly levelled at myself and my colleagues, when we ask for questions, after slogging for a couple of days on a LARSP course, or the like. It is the most dispiriting and dangerous of criticisms, because of course it is a non-criticism. It is not the fault of clinical linguists that their analyses are time-consuming. There is one reason, and only one reason, for the relative complexity and protractedness of such analyses, and that is that phonetic and linguistic handicap is a complex, multi-faceted and variable phenomenon. It is only natural for Ts with heavy caseloads or pupil ratios to demand analytic procedures which are as short and as simple as possible— but the operative words are *as possible*. There are limits beyond which it would be unwise to go, where a procedure would cease to be illuminating and become unreliable. And all linguistically based procedures which have so far been devised have, in the absence of empirical research which might indicate the nature of these limits, erred on the side of caution. You would not thank me if, following this chapter, I presented a quick, ten-minute grammatical analysis, which would enable you to state the obvious, and carry your understanding of your patients or pupils not a whit further forward. But the corollary follows: if you want understanding, insight and remedial confidence, time must be spent. Such prizes are not glibly won.

It is certainly true that the various components of a linguistic approach to handicap demand an outlay of time on T's part which is far above that which would normally be provided on the basis of

traditional practice. While it is possible to do certain types of
analyses on certain types of P in an hour or so, anything at all
complex will regularly require a commitment of a half-day or a
whole day. An initial sample has to be transcribed, analysed,
written up; remediation has to be devised, carried out, and the
results re-analysed; and the cycle may need to begin again. The
greatest outlay of time is in fact on the first of these: the
transcription. Whether it is a phonetic, phonological, orthographic, prosodic or other transcription, or some combination,
this is where the bulk of T's time is going to go. If done well, it is
neither mechanical nor boring. Anyone who has taken the trouble
to write down P's speech accurately and comprehensively knows
how illuminating an exercise it can be. When forced to decide
between whether a sound is X or Y, whether a construction is one
sentence or two, whether enough contextual information is provided to enable an utterance to be interpreted—such experiences
shed fresh light on the inadequacy or instability of P's linguistic
resources. Nor is it a job which can or should be left to an
unsupervised Other, such as a department secretary. A person
untrained in speech transcription simply does not have the ability
to produce the level of accuracy required even for an orthographic
transcription, lacking any special phonetic features. Such a person
inevitably normalizes—even normal speech gets normalized (by
filling out elisions and ellipses, and silently correcting 'incorrect'
usages)—and abnormal speech can be totally misrepresented. The
work has always got to be meticulously checked, and one ends up
using far more time than one hoped to save in the first place! The
task of transcription is far too important to be farmed out. A
transcription, once made, is going to be referred to again and
again; the same transcription might have to serve as the basis for a
prosodic, grammatical, semantic, sociolinguistic or other analysis.
Often, it is not possible to foresee, in making the transcription,
what uses it will one day be put to. So transcribers have just got to
be able to guarantee its accuracy and comprehensiveness, to the
best of their ability. To know that, in a particular ten minutes,
everything P did, linguistically, is down on paper, provides an
empirical datum whose value cannot be underestimated. Transcriptional time is time well-spent. On it, the whole foundation of

our analytic edifice stands.

So, in answer to the question 'How do we justify such an expenditure of time?' my answer is two-fold. First, there is often no alternative: especially in the more complex cases, the limitations of the traditional approach have left T in a position where it is unclear what might be done, and where the only chance to develop a principled therapy or teaching programme is after an appropriately detailed analysis has been made. Secondly, the question of time has to be seen in the long term, and weighed against the criteria of success—in most cases, quantifiable and explicable progress; but in the absence of progress, the confidence that comes from *knowing* that no-one else could have done better. A day devoted to linguistic analysis early on in a case may seem trivial by comparison with the overall amount of time devoted to a patient in subsequent months. And how much time might not be saved by a better distribution of time and resources in the early stages of assessment? There will never be enough time to do everything. 'The days needed 36 hours at least', wrote Elsie Fogerty once, in relation to one period of her life (Cole 1967: p.38). They still do.

The implications of these remarks have yet to be thought through by the remedial professions, and by the bodies which appoint, administer and pay them. On the one hand, there are several clear statements among the various government reports and professional syllabuses that some kind of clinical linguistic analysis is an essential feature of training and professional expertise; on the other hand, no-one has attempted to take the time factor into account in carrying out job-analyses of clinical or teaching practice, with reference to the number of Ps requiring help. The recommendations of the Quirk Report (1972), for example, suggested an aim of 3,500 therapists in Britain, to cope with the current needs of the time (7.28); but current need was defined in terms of the numbers needing treatment, and not in terms of quality of service. 'Case-load', for the Quirk Report, was 'the number of patients on the therapist's treatment and observation register at any one time' (7.24). The examples given 'assume that the necessary paper work, discussions, administrative duties and so on are fitted in as opportunity arises' (7.25). But in the same report, the whole academic foundation of the subject in the UK was in the process of change: 'the would-be practitioner of therapy . . . must in future regard language as the central core of his basic discipline' (6.60), and the teaching of linguistics, the science of language, became a formal part of the speech therapy syllabus two years later. But now, having taught new generations of speech therapists (and several of the old) to do some linguistic analyses, the conflict becomes apparent. These analyses are central to professional expertise, and cannot be lumped together with paperwork, administrative duties, and the like. So how does this affect the notion of case load? My impression is that, if all speech therapists were by some magic to begin doing appropriate linguistic analyses of their patients tomorrow, the effect would be an immediate halving (at least) of their case load. To have anticipated the real effects of their recommendations on language analysis, the Quirk Report should have aimed, not for a doubling, but for a *quadrupling* of speech therapists in subsequent years.

The choice at both individual and administrative levels is clear. If the quality of the service to individual patients is to improve, then *either* this has to be at the expense of quantity of service throughout the community (with some patients not being seen at all, or being seen less often) *or* more therapists have to be employed to make good the deficiency. What is the point of spending hundreds of hours in training students in sophisticated techniques of language analysis—techniques which are of undoubted benefit to the patients—that the system will not allow them to use? It is this sense of frustration which is so often voiced these days. Times have changed, with the new training courses. A new generation of therapists has emerged who do not have to be convinced of the desirability or efficacy of clinical linguistic techniques. It is part of their intellectual and professional make-up to think in these terms. But they are then faced with a political, administrative and economic system which has not come to grips with modern research realities. It is always saddening to hear Ts say they have not been able to do what they wanted with a patient, because of pressure of time. But the solution to this problem is not to water down the intellectual basis of their professionalism, by failing to acquire, or use whenever possible, the relevant analytical knowledge; it is rather to press politically for more opportunities to use that knowledge routinely. Imagine the outcry if a doctor or surgeon proceeded to treat a patient without having done the relevant tests, on grounds of time! Either time would be found, extra staff would be appointed, or of course waiting lists would get longer. The solutions are administrative, not intellectual; and one comes to respect a profession which does not demean its intellectual integrity by accepting a poorer standard of service for administrative reasons. Nor is this problem restricted to speech therapy: the profession of remedial language teaching is an infant, compared to speech therapy, but already the same frustrations are in evidence there, with teachers complaining about the lack of time in which to analyse their pupils' problems.

A responsible attitude to data analysis is a *sine qua non* of progress in the field of remedial language studies, and I certainly do not see the time-consuming nature of some clinical linguistic analyses as an insurmountable barrier. Of course, none of this removes the responsibility from the linguist to devise procedures which are as simple and convenient to use as is commensurate with accuracy and illumination. But everyone must remember the limits referred to above: a procedure, if it becomes too short or simple, becomes unreliable and unilluminating, because it fails to discriminate Ps, or stages of development within individual Ps. Clinical linguists who want to be helpful will always attempt to keep within these limits, and wield Occam's razor at every opportunity. They, as much as anyone, are aware of the problem of time: there are only 24 hours in their, as well as T's, day. It is therefore always infuriating when people in effect criticize clinical linguistics for the unsatisfactory state of affairs, by intimating that it is the analytic procedures themselves which are to blame for the shortage of time.

This is where the 'teeth', referred to in the title of this chapter, enter the argument. I bare mine. But I was not thinking of my own teeth when I decided on this title; I was thinking of Ts' teeth, in the metaphorical sense, as illustrated by such orthodontic metaphors as *put teeth into* (=increase the effectiveness of), *set one's teeth* (= to become resolute) and *show one's teeth* (= to exhibit anger). How may effectiveness be realistically increased, given the constraints on time and numbers which exist? I would be sceptical of any solution which simply proposed 'more speech therapists', 'more teachers'. It is not just a matter of numbers; it is also a matter of the best use of available resources. Having been involved in courses in many parts of the world, I am struck, first and foremost, by the enormous duplication of effort which takes place in assessment procedures, teaching materials and research projects. I do not know how many articulation tests there are, or how many packs of cards which provide pictures of contexts for teaching prepositions; but I do know that there are extensive similarities between the various examples of each genre, such that there is often little to choose between them. And published examples pale alongside the hundreds of privately produced charts, word-lists (such as lists of minimal pairs, for teaching pronunciation) and other documents which individual Ts have spent hours constructing for themselves. Many of these ideas are extremely ingenious and successful. For instance, I saw a device in a Hertfordshire clinic once, which had been designed to provide some visual reinforcement for Subject-Verb-Object clauses. It was a kind of cash-register which, when the keys were pressed, produced SVO pictures of different kinds. Some months later, I saw a very similar invention in Birmingham. Each had taken its inventor hours of labour. How much time is lost, in aggregate, I wonder, due to this process of simultaneous creation? Or again, when the terminology project outlined above was begun, several people wrote to me to say that they belonged to a 'terminology group' in their own locality. They were wanting to systematize the terminology used in their area, but after several meetings they had got into trouble. It is not difficult to see why, in the light of our own experience. But are terminological issues the kind of thing on which time can be profitably spent at local level? It is not difficult to accumulate examples of this kind, where the participants themselves are in doubt about the value of the exercise; nor is it difficult to add further examples, from different areas, where doubts have been expressed about whether the best use is being made of T's time—the therapist who is required to do general clerical duties, or the teacher who is required to do dinner-duty, to take two much-discussed instances.

In the end, it seems to me, the question of time reduces to the question of professionalism. So many of the arguments for and against the term *speech therapy*, in recent debates, were really addressing the question of whether that term did justice to what the job was actually about. But that is a defensive attitude, born of lack of confidence. Real professionals, deep down, do not care a jot what they are called, because they know that what really counts is the authority and specialized knowledge they possess, and to which they or their colleagues have helped to contribute. I sometimes wonder if all the time that has been spent on the name of the profession (and not only in the United Kingdom) had been devoted instead to the writing-up of research reports on Ps, which policy would have been more effective, in the long term, in improving the status of speech therapists in the eyes of others? But here, as in other areas of remedial language work, there seems to be a general lack of a research motivation or initiative at grass-roots level. There is a common reluctance to think beyond the needs of one's individual patients or pupils to the needs of the handicapped population at large. It is a reluctance which stems from a belief that research is for others, for the experts, for those with special training. But research is not the prerogative of a cadre of experts alone. Every new P, in our present state of knowledge, is a research problem of considerable potential interest. Everyone has something they can contribute, by way of observation and description. And for the more advanced work, research training is now obtainable, for those who desire it. It is sometimes said, in relation to speech therapy in the UK, that the new degrees will provide the required change of direction. There is a lot of professional status bound up in a four-year honours degree, and it is a source of satisfaction to see the respect which the new degrees generate among those outside. But it is not something new graduates can do alone. The new generation needs clinical guidance, as well as training in research design, and in the provision of this guidance, the older members of the profession continue to have a crucial, collaborative role. It should never be a question of new versus old, in working with language handicap: it should be new alongside old, if the confident professionalism I am referring to is to become established.

I am struck, finally, by an analogy between the current state of research into language handicap and the state of pathological medicine at the turn of the century. The history of the pathological laboratory has yet to be written, but its development seems to have been a long, slow process. Less than 100 years ago, doctors had to carry out their own pathological analysis, in their own back rooms. Reports of the time frequently complain about pressure of time. In a sense, the present-day speech therapists and remedial language teachers are in the position of these old doctors, having to do their own pathological analysis of speech samples. I would like to think there will come a day when much of the mechanical load will be taken off T's back, by the provision of automatic analysis techniques—techniques of analysis using microprocessors, techniques of remediation using interactive instrumentation. There are promising signs, but the optimal situation will not come about until the basic research position is more advanced than it is at present. As so often, the hardware is ahead of the software. The machines will lighten the load, when we have first told the machines what to do—and this is where we are not.

So the priorities continue to be specialization, research, writing at grass-roots level. Could every T make it their business to write up one P thoroughly, using some of the standard descriptive techniques available? Could this effort be coordinated in some way so that a data bank or archive could be constituted? Could some of the data be organized for publication in one or other of the series which are searching for good material on linguistic handicap? There are so many possibilities, and some will be discussed further in the following pages. The purpose of the present chapter, however, is not to investigate solutions: it is to draw attention to a problem, an unhealthy excess of zeal for terminological matters, given the present primitive state of our knowledge of clinical linguistic symptomatology. I have argued that these priorities must be reversed, and that time must be found to enable specialists in language handicap to practise what is preached. The solution is in T's own teeth, for it will take every effort to fight for what is required. But preaching alone will not exorcize the terminological demon. Only good clinical linguistic practice will do that.

2

Clinical linguistics

Clinical linguistics is the application of the theories, methods and findings of linguistics (including phonetics) to the study of those situations where language handicaps are diagnosed and treated. It is a moot point whether 'clinical' is the most appropriate term. It is chosen because the settings which first attracted detailed linguistic study were medical, and the context of intervention was the speech therapy clinic. In recent years, remedial language work has come to be carried on in non-medical settings—most notably, in educational, social and psychological contexts, where the concept of 'clinical' is less appropriate. A case might thus be made for devising a more general label for remedial language studies. The term 'remedial' has in fact itself been proposed ('remedial linguistics') but this suffers from the double criticism of being both too broad (for some people, it would include work on foreign languages) and too narrow (for others, it would relate primarily to the underachieving population of secondary schools; see further, Chapter 5). There does not seem to be an appropriate general term, which cuts across the clinical and educational domains, to refer to all the categories of language handicap, from disorder to underachievement. I often use 'remedial' in this book, but not without risk, because of its ambiguity. The irony of it. When one does want a term, there is none to be found. I can hear the terminology demon laughing from here. So it goes.

The orientation of the above definition should also be noted. It may be contrasted with the approach of many neurolinguists, for example, who study clinical language data in order to gain insights into linguistic or neurological theory. This too might be referred to under the heading of 'clinical linguistics', but it is not the main orientation of this book. For me, clinical linguistics is first and foremost a branch of applied linguistics, though one about which it is difficult to generalize, perhaps because there are so few clinical linguists around. What follows is therefore inevitably a personal account, based on the kind of clinical analyses in which I have been involved in recent years.

To apply linguistics in the domain of language pathology requires that the linguist be aware of what counts as clinical criteria. When linguists are not aware of these criteria, they run the risk of their observations, no matter how well-intentioned, being inapplicable, for a variety of reasons. It is therefore necessary to begin with an explicit statement of what Ts feel to be needed, in order to obtain progress in their field. Such points as the following have been routinely cited in clinical discussions, and they provide the perspective within which a linguist can work: the cardinal importance of P's remediation as the goal of the exercise; the need to integrate the range of intermediate clinical skills (such as screening, assessment and diagnosis) in relation to this goal; and the desire to integrate the methods and findings of the various remedial professions. Above all, I note the concern to develop explicitly principled methods of intervention, which can provide a basis for explaining both the successes and the failures in working with Ps, and thus a more conscious professionalism. Clinical confidence comes when Ts are in a position to verify the efficacy of their intervention strategies. Clinical insight comes when Ts' training enables them to see a pattern in a mass of data, and to make predictions about P's progress in response to teaching strategies. It is in relation to these two aims—clinical insight and confidence—that the application of linguistics can make its main contribution (see further, Crystal 1981: Chapter 1).

The specific contributions of clinical linguistics can be summarized under eight headings:

(a) the clarification of areas of confusion in the use of the traditional metalanguage of language pathology (cf. Chapter 1);

(b) the systematic description of P linguistic behaviour, T

linguistic behaviour, and their interaction;

(c) the analysis of these descriptions, in order to demonstrate the extent to which P is operating systematically;

(d) the classification of P linguistic behaviours, as part of the process of differential diagnosis;

(e) the assessment of P linguistic behaviours, by demonstrating P's position on scales of approximation to linguistic norms;

(f) the formulation of hypotheses for remediation of P's linguistic behaviour;

(g) the evaluation of the outcome of these hypotheses, as teaching proceeds;

(h) the evaluation of the remedial strategies used in the intervention, insofar as linguistic variables are involved.

What has to be appreciated is that, while it is the later tasks that are central to T's purpose, these are wholly dependent on the earlier tasks in the list. Remediation presupposes assessment, which presupposes analysis, which presupposes description. Without an adequate description, accordingly, Ts cannot guarantee the objective basis of their work. I do not deny the value of the intuitive approach of the experienced T, but if this approach on occasion does not work, or if Ts want to be able to explain the basis of their successes and failures, the need for systematic description and analysis becomes paramount, as a foundation of enquiry.

This is where clinical linguistic studies present something of a paradox, at the present time. On the one hand, linguists have available a range of analytical instrumentation and descriptive techniques whose power far exceeds that currently available in a field such as neurology, even allowing for advances in nuclear magnetic resonance, and the availability of post mortem as a check on hypotheses. I can describe almost every aspect of the stream of speech in minute detail, and in a short time can accumulate far more acoustic, articulatory or auditorily transcribed data than I have time to analyse. On the other hand, the use of these techniques for the linguistic description of clinical cases is far from routine, and in no way matches the level of detailed presentation which we associate with the medical studies of the past 100 years. There are several published accounts of aspects of

Ps' linguistic disability, as already suggested in Chapter 1, but I have not found an account in which the *whole* of someone's residual linguistic skills is presented—phonetic, phonological (non-segmental as well as segmental), grammatical, semantic, pragmatic, etc.— with proper attention paid to comprehension as well as production. There are many partial studies and illustrations, of course, which give sample utterances, snippets of dialogue, test results and linguistic observations; and these help to build up a clinical characterization of a condition, and provide input for the formulation of theories and therapies of linguistic handicap. But the goal of a comprehensive and precise description of P's linguistic strengths and weaknesses is still far from routine, and is usually missing from published accounts of research investigations or of therapeutic practice. It is not even obvious what form such routine case-descriptions should take, if they were to be published.

Something needs to be done. Clinical language studies desperately need to develop a tradition of clinical reference, so that standard descriptions of P syndromes become available, along with samples of data—though without requiring, one imagines, the role of the post mortem! Not only would students benefit from such a development (cf. p.18), researchers would benefit also, in that they would be able to develop a tradition of routine awareness of classical cases, such as we encounter in medical science, where everyone knows 'Broca's patient', for example. But so far there are no equivalents to Broca or Wernicke in the clinical linguistic field, with the splendid exception of Roman Jakobson.

The reason for the paradox, I do not doubt, is the paucity of people working in clinical linguistics, as a result of which even the most basic of findings have made little impact on the awareness of those working in associated disciplines. It is still routine to encounter in fields such as speech therapy, psychology or neurology the use of descriptive terminology which, from a linguistic point of view, is vague and inadequate. Terms such as *agrammatism, paraphasia*, and the like—notwithstanding their frequent use—are, from a linguistic point of view, only the most elementary of approximations, lacking any real precision. Neurologists interested in aphasia would be most unhappy if one began to refer to areas of the brain using such labels as 'the front', 'the left side towards the back', instead of the more accurate terminology available. In like manner, linguists would prefer to use a more detailed descriptive apparatus for the presentation of clinical cases.

'Empirical work must come first.' It is discomfiting, but salutary to recall this quotation—discomfiting, because it was a remark of Hughlings Jackson, made in the 1880s at a British Medical Association meeting, and the remark is as apposite today as it was a century ago. So much has happened in the interim, and yet there still remains a pressing need for comprehensive and precise descriptions of the linguistic behaviour of all Ps—not only the aphasic ones—at a level of detail which would be considered routine in, say, human anatomy or physiology. Some years ago, this demand was voiced primarily with reference to questions of diagnosis and assessment; more recently, with reference to procedures of treatment and rehabilitation; more recently still, with the problem of how to evaluate therapy or teaching. Indeed, these days the demand for an initial linguistic description seems to take on the status of an axiom, in the accounts of many scholars. For example, in the introductory chapter of a recent volume on aphasia therapy (Code and Muller 1983), the editors remark: 'a description of the patient's communicative abilities along linguistic parameters would appear to be essential before treatment can be planned.' And in the concluding chapter to the same volume, Coltheart remarks: 'any study intending to obtain information about the efficacy of any form of treatment should begin with the assembling of a good description of the patient' (Chapter 18). In another recent review, the author states: 'a detailed analysis of a patient's spontaneous speech is the first step in planning a treatment programme' (Ludlow 1981: p.163). Comments of this kind are widespread, in the aphasia literature, and in relation to other syndromes, which makes the complete absence of comprehensive descriptions all the more noticeable, and regrettable.

The need for descriptive statements is not motivated solely by the demands of therapy, but also by the requirements of differential diagnosis. It is nowadays something of a truism to point to the terminological uncertainty and the competing typologies which characterize the field of aphasiology, for example. 'There is still no universally agreed definition of aphasia,' complains Lesser on her opening page (1978: p.1), and, after reviewing various syndromes, she concludes: 'it would be a mistake to give the impression that these syndromes are easily recognisable in a clinical population' (*ibid.*: p. 18). Whurr (1982) begins similarly, with reference to typology: 'there is still no universally agreed classification. Terminological confusion exists, due, in part, to the multidisciplinary interest in the subject (clinical, physiological and behavioural), but also due to the diversity of philosophical and psychological theories on which much of the work has been based,' and she concludes: 'In the absence of such descriptive statements, the traditional aphasiological foci of attention on matters of definition, diagnosis and classification seem positively misguided' (1982: pp.239, 255). The role of accurate linguistic description of P behaviour as a means of resolving these problems has long been appreciated: Jakobson, for instance, argued the importance of the point for thirty years (see, for example, Jakobson 1954). But as recently as 1980, he still found it necessary to say: 'the further development of linguistic enquiry into aphasia demands a greater concentration on the description and classification of the purely verbal syndromes' (1980: p.107). Jakobson's own pioneering application of linguistic concepts to aphasia is rightly regarded as monumental, but his classifications remain extremely general, and have not, it seems, been followed up with detailed sub-classifications carried out at appropriate linguistic levels, or with applications which have related his intentions to the specific demands of routine clinical practice.

The reasons for the lack of descriptive progress are not hard to find. The task presupposes an adequate descriptive framework, and knowledge of how to use and apply it. Insofar as linguistics is concerned with the provision of descriptive frameworks for language, it has to be pointed out that reasonably comprehensive frameworks have only recently come to be devised, and there are still many gaps which remain to be filled by pure research. Similarly, the training of those people most involved in the study of aphasia, and other syndromes, has until recently lacked components in which such descriptive frameworks are routinely taught and practised. It is only since 1974, after all, that a course on linguistic theory and description became an obligatory feature of speech therapy training in the UK; and it is rare indeed to find such a course as part of teacher training in special education. But even in centres where the frameworks are available, and the willingness to learn and use them is present, there are problems, such as the problem of time (Chapter 1). As a result, there is a marked lack of publicly accessible data, and no guarantee that the data which are available have involved the use of the same descriptive framework, to enable comparative statements to be made in a clear and consistent way.

The theoretical framework required to make progress with the descriptive problem has been appreciated for a long time: a model of language which recognizes and interrelates a set of linguistic *levels* — dimensions of linguistic analysis capable of independent study. In relation to aphasiology, the importance of this model is summarized by Jakobson (1980: pp.94-5):

> The question of levels is relevant indeed. Too often, attempts to treat the linguistic aspect of aphasia suffer from inadequate delimitation of the linguistic levels. One could even say that today the most important task in linguistics is to learn how to delimit the levels. . . But in all linguistic questions and especially in the case of aphasia, it is important to approach language and its disruption in the framework of a given level, while remembering at the same time that . . . the totality and the interrelation between the different parts of the totality have to be taken into account.

Reference to at least the main levels of linguistic inquiry is now commonplace in aphasia studies: it seems conventional to recognize the levels of phonology, grammar and semantics (as in Lesser 1978: pp.24ff.; Albert *et al.* 1981: pp.13ff.; Whurr 1982; and many others). But this recognition of the theoretical imortance of the model has not been accompanied by a corresponding readiness to provide descriptions in terms of the model. The idea of levels has proved its worth by providing a framework within which clinical observations can be placed somewhat more neatly than previously, and it has acted as a reminder to clinicians of the potential complexity of language; but in fact hardly any publications illustrate its systematic, detailed descriptive use, and there is a real danger of misleading conclusions being drawn about aphasia, or about any other language handicap, when the limitations of the model fail to be understood, and the notion of level comes to be applied in an oversimplified way.

Before proceeding to discuss the descriptive approach further, accordingly, some cautionary remarks are in order. In particular, it must not be forgotten that the concept of 'level' is a linguistic fiction, with both the number of levels and the nature of their boundaries being the outcome of specific linguistic theories. It is fashionable these days to search for neurological or psychological correlates of linguistic levels, but we do not have to commit ourselves to a 'God's truth' view of these constructs in order to use them, and indeed there are interesting arguments against adopting such a view (as I have discussed elsewhere, Crystal 1982b). The three-level approach, for example, is only one such possibility. There are also two-level models (e.g. form versus meaning, or structure versus use), four-level models (e.g. recognizing a separate level of phonetics alongside phonology, or a level of morphology alongside syntax), five-level models (phonetics/phonology/morphology/syntax/semantics); and so on. In some approaches, different kinds of levels are recognized, as in Halliday's notion of 'inter-levels' (of phonology and semantics), whose role is to relate the primary levels of substance, form and context (Halliday 1961). The linguistics literature has spent a great deal of space considering how levels of analysis are motivated and applied, and it is now generally recognized that levels ought not to be presented as if they had some kind of life of their own, but rather ought to be seen within a particular theoretical frame of reference.

As a brief example of this point, let us consider the enquiry 'Is there a level of prosody?' What has to be appreciated is that there is no single answer to this question. Some approaches see prosody as a sub-level within phonology ('non-segmental' or 'suprasegmental' as opposed to 'segmental' phonology, they would say); some see it as separate from phonology (they would talk about a 'phonological *and* prosodic analysis', for example); others see it as best subsumed under the level of grammar; and there are other possible positions. To choose between these alternatives, we must first know something about the range of forms and functions which are designated by the term 'prosody'—the variations in pitch, loudness, speed and rhythm of speech—and reflect on the extent to which these variations operate in language as do the phonemes or distinctive features of phonology, or the syntactic rules of grammar. Only after we have made a judgement about their linguistic role and significance, will we be able to decide whether to 'promote' them to the status of a linguistic level, and give them some kind of autonomy in our description (see further, Crystal 1969: pp.179ff.).

It must be remembered, too, that linguistics is concerned with the properties of language in general (not just English, or modern European languages), and that its models have to be tested against the variety of languages encountered in the world. It is not enough to devise a levels model which works quite well for English, and assume its psycholinguistic or neurolinguistic reality, forgetting that the model may not work so well for structurally unrelated languages (whose speakers nonetheless have to be credited with isomorphic brains). A stroke is no respecter of languages. And aphasia studies must therefore be generalizable in a way that they usually are not. To take just one example, Lesser (1978: p.24) decides that, in her book, 'as is more usual in aphasiology, the term *syntax* will be used to include morphology as well as sentence structure.' Now it is certainly possible to devise a theory in which a level of morphology has no separate representation (generative grammar, for instance), and such a theory does not do too much harm to the facts of English, where inflectional endings are few. But it is most unlikely that such a theory would do justice to aphasic behaviour in, say, Turkish or Japanese (which are agglutinating languages, with complex word-structure), or Arabic or Greek (which are languages with a complex inflectional system). In such cases, the morphological component of the description would be so important that it would have to be recognized in our general approach as a major level, and not be swallowed up as a junior aspect of the syntax. And similar issues are raised in relation to any of the other linguistic levels.

A further cautionary observation relates to the notion of 'autonomy' of levels. As Jakobson and many other theoreticians have emphasized: 'The various levels of language are autonomous. [But] Autonomy doesn't mean isolationism; all levels are interrelated' (Jakobson 1980: p.94). And indeed, the convenience of a framework in which we are permitted to study a single aspect of linguistic form or function to the exclusion of others must not be allowed to obscure the artefactual nature of this manoeuvre, nor to minimize the importance of expounding the nature of the relationships which obtain between levels, and which define the language system as a whole. Points of contact between levels are frequently noted in clinical investigation, in fact—for example, the functional load of the phoneme /s/ at the grammatical level (where it realises plurality, possession, 3rd person present tense, etc.), or the use of rising intonation as an alternative to syntactic forms of question, or the way in which lexical problems interfere with the construction of sentences (as in so-called 'word-finding' difficulties). Nor are these isolated topics: in principle, *all* descriptive statements made at a given level must be related to the corresponding statements made at other levels, the interactions noted, and some kind of integrated account arrived at. We must beware of Humpty Dumpty syndrome. We should never take language apart without the intention and ability to put it back together again.

The importance of transcription

An integrated transcription in terms of levels is an important goal of clinical studies, but it cannot even begin to be achieved without a firm transcriptional foundation, and this is usually lacking. As already emphasized in Chapter 1 (p.23), whenever we obtain a sample from P for linguistic study (whether of spontaneous speech, test results, reading aloud, or whatever), the first step should be to make a good transcription of it. But what does 'good' mean in this context? A good transcription, in essence, is an account of the sample which makes it unnecessary to refer back to the tape from which it derived. It 'replaces' the tape, in the sense that any analysts trained in the transcriptional conventions can read the transcription and 'hear' what was said as clearly as if they were listening to the tape itself. They can then use the transcription as a check on the transcriber's descriptive claims. By contrast, if a transcription is unclear, partial or inconsistent, it becomes impossible to verify anything. Now, few transcriptions ever reach the ideal state of autonomy, and achieve a life of their own; but we all have to strive to attain a reasonable level of accuracy and consistency. Unfortunately, transcriptions of handicapped speech are rarely complete, and are usually ambiguous in the claims they make.

To illustrate this, let us look at the kind of transcription generally encountered in published work on aphasia. The following example is taken from one of the pioneering papers on the linguistic analysis of this syndrome (Goodglass 1968: p.178):

> Yes .... ah .... Monday ... ah ... Dad and Peter Hogan, and Dad ... ah ... Hospital ... and ah ... Wednesday ... Wednesday, nine o'clock and ah Thursday ... ten o'clock ah doctors ... two ... two ... an doctors and ... ah ... teeth ... yah. And a doctor ... an girl ... and gums, and I.

It is impossible to derive from such a transcription a clear auditory impression of how P must have spoken this utterance. The punctuation is partly conventional (periods and commas), partly unconventional (the use of triple dots, but in two cases the use of quadruple dots). Are the dots intended to represent a *system* of pauses, in the sense that all triple dots are the same length? What exact value has the comma, in relation to the other punctuation features? What was it in the data that led the analyst to use a period after *yah* and not a comma or triple dot? Or (to move to lexico-grammatical issues), what is the evidence to support the transcription of *an* in two places, instead of *and*? Does the fact that *Hospital* is written with a capital letter mean that the analyst is seeing this word as a proper noun, or as the beginning of a new sentence, or both? A transcription of this kind raises many such questions, none of which is trivial, for analytic decisions will later be made to depend on them. If we wish to measure the length of this P's sentences, for instance, the decisions which led the transcriber to assign periods will be crucial.

There seems to have been no change in this kind of loose transcriptional practice since the 1960s. Ludlow (1981: p.151), for example, illustrates the following Broca P's utterance:

Me ... my wife ... went ... school, no, speech, speech, speech therapy. Oh, I don't know, I went ... and work, work.

The same problems recur. Why is there a comma after *school*, and not a period? What motivated the period after *therapy*? Why no period after *know*?

The use of punctuation, supplemented by an arbitrary and idiosyncratic list of graphic devices, seems to be standard practice in aphasia studies still, as in most other fields of language handicap, and it will not do. Such an approach leaves out far too much relevant information—information which is prerequisite for anyone wishing to sharpen their instruments for diagnosis and assessment, or to improve their techniques of remediation. Most obviously, these transcriptions omit to tell us anything about the intonation, stress, rhythm and other prosodic and paralinguistic features of spoken language—features which are central to our understanding of the organization and progress of aphasic speech. Indeed, it is the particular combination of one of these features (stress) with certain word clusters which, in Goodglass' view, 'forms the essential feature of the agrammatism of Broca's aphasia' (1968: p.206)—and we might note in this respect Lesser's balanced discussion (1978: pp.182ff.). But if this is the case, we would at least expect aphasic transcriptions to contain stress marks, to enable researchers to check the hypothesis, and this is not routinely done.

But it is not simply a matter of stress. The multiple functions of intonation in the organization and processing of speech are strongly implicated in the search for an explanation of aphasic disturbance. Is each word in a given sequence spoken with a separate intonation unit (a 'word-at-a-time' intonation)? Or do the words group themselves intonationally (and rhythmically) in certain ways? If the latter, the particular groupings can tell us a great deal about the way P is processing language, and where his difficulties lie. An example is the abnormal chunking introduced by prosody into one of Mr J's sentences (Crystal, Fletcher and Garman 1976: pp.177ff.). Mr J would say, at a certain stage in his treatment:

the bòy is/ . èating a/ . àpple/*

Later, he was able to say:

the bòy/ is . èating/ a . àpple/

still somewhat hesitant, but at least now the main prosodic units correspond to the main grammatical elements of the sentence. To show this improvement, we require a transcription in which at least the tone unit boundaries, tonicity and nuclear tone type are marked, along with stress and pause conventions, where needed.

The kind of transcription illustrated here is of course still only a crude level of phonological representation. To capture the whole range of non-segmental phonological features available in a language, a much more detailed level of transcription is required, in which such variables as increases and decreases of tempo and loudness, alterations in the pitch range of stretches of utterance, rhythmical variations and the many kinds of vocal paralinguistic effect (e.g. breathy, creaky, nasal, or tense tones of voice) are taken into account. The level of detail of such a transcription has been illustrated elsewhere, for normal varieties of English (see footnote), where it is possible to identify the salient phonological characteristics of, say, a sermon, or a sports commentary, or everyday conversation, using such a combination of variables. It is my view that the non-segmental variability of language handi-

---

* / marks tone-unit boundaries; ` represents a falling tone; . represents a brief pause; ' represents a stressed syllable; all other syllables are unstressed. These conventions are taken from the transcriptional system presented in Crystal (1969), used in full in Crystal and Davy (1969), and in simplified form in Crystal, Fletcher and Garman (1976) and elsewhere.

cap is no less complex than that encountered in other varieties of a language, and deserves a comparably serious treatment. This is most obviously the case for the more 'fluent' kinds of aphasia, where variations in pitch range, loudness and speed are often important cues to our awareness of P's comprehension and control of what he says. Thus one P (Mrs W) used to produce fairly well-formed sentences, consisting of main clause and subordinate clause, as follows:

well I used to go down there whenever I could you see

which, lacking any prosodic transcription, tells us nothing about her problems of expression and her listener's problems of comprehension. In fact, what Mrs W said was:

'well I 'used to 'go down thére/''when' ever I còuld you sée/'
'low,piano,allegro'   'crescendo,ascending,lento'

where the inverted commas indicate that the first, main clause was spoken in a low-pitched, quiet and rapid tone of voice, and the second, subordinate clause was spoken with the voice level increasing and slowing. In short, the overall auditory effect was something like:

.... whenever I could you see.

This consistent obscuring of the main clauses in Mrs W's speech was an important feature of her assessment, and an early target for remediation. Similar forms of prosodic complexity can be demonstrated for other types of aphasia—for example, the variations in the tempo of utterance of syllables and segments in 'nonfluent' speech.

It should be noted, at this point, that my requirement of a reasonably full prosodic and paralinguistic transcription of language handicapped speech is not an abnormally strong one: it is no greater than what I would expect as a foundation for the description of any sample of spoken language. But in the case of many kinds of handicap, and certainly in the case of aphasia, the requirement has an added significance, in that it is a prerequisite for an adequate symptomatology (cf. p.17). I take it as axiomatic that an aim of language pathology is a comprehensive statement of clinical symptoms. And in a case such as aphasiology, it is often said, impressionistically, that the prosody is disturbed. But little effort has been made to build an appropriate bridge between these last two sentences. Thus, for example, in a recent synthesis representing the influential Boston approach, we have an account of Melodic Intonation Therapy, and an interesting case report, on the one hand (Albert *et al.* 1981: pp.147ff.); but on the other hand, the authors do not give any intonational transcription of their P's speech, and in their introduction, the section on 'linguistic aspects of dysphasia testing' makes no mention of intonation or prosody at all (pp.12ff.). There are several valuable hypotheses about prosody in aphasia, and several experimental studies (cf. Lesser's review, 1978: pp.28-9, 182-5), but there is a remarkable lack of naturalistic empirical data on the point. We urgently need descriptions of Ps' prosodic and paralinguistic features, both in a range of linguistic settings, and longitudinally; equally, we need similar transcriptions of the prosody and paralanguage of Ps' interlocutors, the prosodic character of whose stimuli exercises so much influence on Ps' response (see further p.72).

Segmental phonological transcriptions of spontaneous or elicited speech samples (that is, of the vowel/consonant sequences which constitute the 'verbal' aspect of utterance), although somewhat more familiar than prosodic ones, are nonetheless by no means routinely made. Here too, we encounter the need for an objective transcription, not simply to provide the input for the description of P's articulation problems (if any), but to provide a data-base for the verification of grammatical and semantic hypotheses. Even the most experienced analysts have to be on their guard against reading in grammatical or semantic information into what they hear on a tape. A phonetic sequence such as [ən] could be a realization of *and, an, in, on,* or other words; and if contextual clues are ambiguous or absent, as is often the case in Ps' conversations about themselves or their backgrounds, what justification has T got for assigning one rather than another of these interpretations to the sounds in question? In the transcript illustrated on p.40, for example, what grounds were there for a transcription of *an doctors* and *an girl*, as opposed to, say, *and doctors ... and girl*? Was there something in the phonetics which motivated Goodglass' decision? If the phonetic evidence was [ən], it would have been better to transcribe it thus, to enable other analysts to judge the matter for themselves, and perhaps argue for alternative grammatico-lexical interpretations. One of my own commonest problems, in this respect, is what to do with a final [s] following a noun, in non-fluent speech. P talks about a car and then says *brother*[s]: does he mean *brothers* (plural), *brother's* (possessive), *brothers'*, or *brother's* (i.e. 'brother is' or 'brother has')? It is easy to underestimate the amount of analytical indeterminacy in the description of disordered speech.

Indeed, it is only in recent years that the concept of phonetic indeterminacy has received investigation at all, in the attempts by various groups to set up new conventions for phonetic transcription, in which uncertainty is formally recognized (Grunwell *et al.* 1980). I strongly approve of this development. The clean-looking phonetic transcriptions of Ps' speech, which look as if the sounds have been articulated by a radio announcer, are disturbing idealizations. It may seem like stating the obvious, but if Ps have the kind of abnormal pronunciation which requires a transcription, then this will mean that they will be difficult to understand, and therefore transcribe. It is this last clause which is not so obvious. Only very rarely is it easy to transcribe abnormal pronunciation, because of the uncertainties over degree of voicing, aspiration, place of articulation (especially regarding vowels), and so on. A transcription needs to reflect these realities, and transcribers need to learn to realize that problems of transcription are endemic. Many of the problems they have to face are 'not their fault' (though any students reading this must not take it as an excuse to miss the next phonetics ear-training class!). We know from general phonetics that a discrete set of two-dimensionally-defined symbols cannot be imposed without distortion onto a stream of non-discrete, multidimensional sound. But in the context of language handicap, there is more involved than just the general principle. In the phonetic transcription of normal speech, we learn to tolerate the arbitrariness (though the limitation of systems such as the IPA regularly provokes debate in phonetics journals), because the phonological analysis is well understood. In the case of disordered speech, we cannot be so tolerant, because it is the nature of the phonological system which we are trying to demonstrate. We therefore need to be as faithful to the data as our ears (or instrumentation) will allow. And this means being ready to recognize when a sound is wholly or partly untranscribable. The most useful symbol of all is ○. Placed around another symbol, it means, in effect, 'I'm not sure about this one.' ⓟ means 'I think it was [p], but I'm not sure.' ⓢ means 'I think it was a stop, but I'm not sure.' ⓒ means 'I think it was a consonant, but I'm not sure which one.' And ○ alone means 'I think it was a sound, but I'm not sure which one.' Since these symbols were introduced, I have found myself using them increasingly, and they have enlarged immeasurably the meaningfulness and reliability of my transcriptions. No longer do I have to cross my fingers and opt for a symbol (which, even with a set of diacritics, implies a definite sound identification), or clutter up the page with question marks (always ambiguous, in retrospect, as there is nothing in the question mark to indicate what the basis of the auditory problem was). These symbols have taken a lot of the guilt out of phonetic transcription.

Organizing linguistic observations

A reliable transcription is the fuel which drives a model of language organized in terms of levels. But it is not really possible to appreciate the model's organizing power until we can place it in a broader theoretical context, for which we need to make some reference to the semiotic perspective in the analysis of human communicative behaviour.

Semiotics has received many definitions, but the one which I think is most relevant for present purposes is 'patterned communications in all modalities' (Sebeok, Hayes and Bateson 1964: p.5). The approach stresses 'the interactional and communicative context of the human use of signs, and the way in which these are organised in transactional systems involving sight, hearing, touch, smell, taste'. From the point of view of language handicap, such a broad perspective is to be welcomed, as it prompts us to remember in our enquiry the potential communicative role of *all* sensory modalities, including those (such as touch) whose relevance has been underestimated, and those (such as smell and taste) whose relevance is generally ignored—though we can hardly doubt the importance to P of the 'passive' signals he receives through these modalities. However, only the first three of the five modalities have received a great deal of study, and become institutionalized in the academic literature, as can be seen from Figure 1, which recognizes the domains of linguistics, kinesics and proxemics.

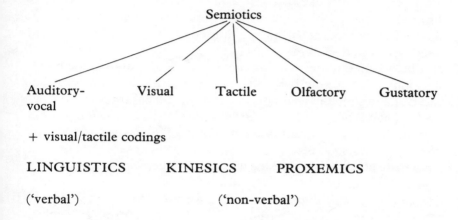

Figure 1   The semiotic frame

The use of the auditory-vocal channel as a means of human communication (i.e. 'speech', or, more precisely, 'spoken language') is pre-eminently the concern of linguistics. But other visual or tactile 'codings' based on speech would also be subsumed under the heading of linguistic study—first-order codes, such as writing ('written language'), or second-order codes, such as finger-spelling. More complex signing systems, too, have to be allowed for: those which have a direct relationship with the patterns of spoken or written language (such as the Paget-Gorman Signing System) and those which do not (such as British Sign Language).

Under the heading of *kinesics* is included the study of facial expression and bodily gesture—purely visual systems of communication, lacking any derivational connection with spoken or written language, and lacking the scope and productivity that we associate with deaf signing systems. *Proxemics* studies the tactile medium of communication (as in hand-shaking, etc.), but the term reflects more a research interest in such matters as the way variations in physical distance between human beings can be used as a communicative signal. Again, a distinction must be drawn between the everyday use of proxemic behaviour, which is quite limited in scope, and the contrived use of such behaviour in specially designed signalling systems (such as the Tadoma system used with the deaf-blind).

The distinction between linguistic behaviour, on the one hand, and kinesic/proxemic behaviour, on the other, is similar to that often encountered in psychology between 'verbal communication' and 'non-verbal communication'. But the verbal/non-verbal terminology obscures a matter which is of some importance for clinical language studies, so I shall not use it here—namely, that under the heading of language we need to recognize the important features of prosody (cf. p.37), which are patently vocal, but not verbal. No binary division does them justice, for at one extreme such features interact closely with the structures of spoken language (in such contexts as stating versus questioning, or focusing attention on particular words in a sentence), and at the other extreme they are used for the communication of emotion, in a similar way to kinesic or proxemic behaviour. Drawing a boundary around the notion of 'language' is always a somewhat arbitrary procedure, as a consequence. It is never wise to be dogmatic over what is or is not 'language'.

Having said this, let me now proceed to be dogmatic by suggesting that there is little to be gained by extending the use of the term 'language' to cover all the domains of semiotic enquiry, as is often done through the use of such expressions as 'body language'. In these expressions, the term has come to be synonymous with 'communication', and a valuable distinction is in danger of being lost. However, clear differences exist between the kind of behaviour demonstrated by the use of spoken/written language and that encountered in the kinesic/proxemic domain. The remarkable *productivity* (or creativity) of the grammar and lexicon of language is one criterion of difference; another is the *dual structure* of language (a level of meaningless units—such as sounds or letters—combining to form a level of meaningful units, such as words and sentences). Yet other criteria have been explored (Hockett 1958, Hockett and Altmann 1968) in support of the conclusion that there are major qualitative differences between spoken/written language, on the one hand, and the various kinds of 'non-verbal' communication, on the other. Concept-based deaf signing systems sit somewhat uneasily between the two, but present-day social attitudes forcefully support their characterization as 'language', and focusing on the dissimilarities between spoken/written language in particular and signing systems in general is nowadays felt to be counter-productive.

We may now focus more precisely on specifically linguistic considerations, within this general semiotic perspective. The first factor to take into account is that all linguistic theories draw a distinction between the structural properties of language and the range of functions to which language can be put. This distinction turns out to be highly relevant when it comes to the investigation of language handicap. On the one hand, there are people whose handicap takes the form of a limitation in their ability to use the structures of spoken/written language; on the other hand, there are those whose control of structure is relatively advanced, but who lack the ability to put these structures to good use in real communicative situations. It is within these two broadly defined areas of *language structure* and *language use* that the various levels of language have come to be routinely identified.

Under the heading of structure, most accounts recognize three main levels: *semantics, grammar*, and the properties of the *transmission system* chosen (i.e. whether spoken, written, or signed). This is not the place to discuss each of these levels in detail, for such an exposition is available elsewhere (e.g. Crystal 1981); but a brief resumé may be helpful to some readers (and those for whom the following paragraphs are redundant may pick up the trail again on p.58). Semantics, first of all, is the study of the way meaning is structured in language. At the most general level, it involves the study of the way we organize the meaning of what we want to say or write into stretches of language (which are often called *discourses* or *texts*), as when we expound a story in a logical way, or maintain a coherent structure in a piece of dialogue. Discourse breakdowns are common in handicapped language, as when questions fail to be answered appropriately, or irrelevant or disjointed remarks are introduced into a conversation. At a more detailed level, semantics involves the study of vocabulary, not just by making lists of words (more precisely, 'lexical items'), but a study of the way in which these items relate to each other and define each other. When we say that *car, automobile* and *old crock* have similar meanings (are synonyms), or that *old* is the opposite of *young* (are antonyms), or that *cow, horse* and *sheep* are all *animals* (more precisely, are hyponyms of *animal*), then we are making statements about the relationships between lexical items. It is the learning of these relationships which constitutes the main task in the acquisition of vocabulary. We cannot assess lexical ability simply by counting the number of words P uses, for two Ps may have similar sizes of vocabulary, but be very different in their awareness of how the lexical items relate to each other. Similarly, teaching procedures need to take into account the structural characteristics of the lexical system (see further, Crystal 1981, 1982a).

The distinction between semantics and grammar can be drawn in the following way. If we have a meaning 'in mind', such as a request to have a locked door opened, there are innumerable ways in which we might express this meaning, using the same vocabulary, and also many ways in which the language does *not* permit us to express this meaning. Among the permitted ways are such sentences as *I need a key to open the door, This door needs a key, If we had a key, we could open the door*, and so on. Among the disallowed sentences are *need I a key this door to open, open could the the door a locked*, and so on. Grammar is the study of sentence structures and sequences, from the viewpoint of which strings of words are acceptable in a language, and how they relate to each other. It is often divided into two sub-fields. *Morphology* is the study of the structure of words, of the way words can be made larger by adding different prefixes and suffixes, and by joining units together in various ways, e.g. *boy/boys, go/going/gone, nation/ nationalize/nationalization*. *Syntax* is the study of the way words are strung together to make up the phrases and sentences of a language, the study of the various patterns of word order and word substitution, and of the kinds of relationship which exist between these patterns. Consider the differences between *The dog chased the man* and *The man chased the dog, Did the man chase the dog?*, and so on. There are obviously rules governing the way in which these sentences relate to each other, and it is the task of syntax to explain what these rules are. Not surprisingly, in view of the complexity involved, grammatical disability is a major feature of most kinds of language handicap. And, as with semantic analysis, simple measures of grammar in terms of sentence length, or the like, will not suffice to capture this complexity: two Ps may have similar sentence lengths, but be vastly different in the kind of grammatical structures they are able to handle (Crystal, Fletcher and Garman 1976: Chapter 1).

Let us now assume that we have a meaning 'in mind', and have decided which sentence pattern to use to express it; there remains the third level of language structure to be taken into account. We have to choose which way to transmit the message, whether in speech or in writing, or using some other coded medium, such as finger-spelling, signing or semaphore. Restricting the case to spoken language, for present purposes, we have to distinguish right away between those properties of the transmission system which are *independent* of a particular language, and those which are *dependent*. The kinds of things which can handicap a person under the first of these headings are very different from those which can handicap him under the second. Unfortunately, the everyday term 'pronunciation' does not make this distinction clear, and so new terminology has to be introduced to handle it. It is now conventional to distinguish, firstly, the range of sounds which the human vocal tract can produce and the human ear perceive—a very great range indeed; and, secondly, the much more restricted range of sounds which actually turn up in a language. The study of the first of these, the general study of human sound-making and sound-reception, is known as *phonetics*.

The study of the second, the sound system of a particular language or language-group, is known as *phonology*.

The relevance of the distinction to handicap is as follows. In the absence of any pathology, all human beings are born with the same capacities for sound in their ears, vocal tracts and brains. Similarly, pathologies of hearing, articulation or nervous system affect speakers all over the world in the same way, regardless of the language community in which they live. A given type of deafness will devastate a member of the English speech community in the same way as it will the French. The nasal resonance of a cleft palate child will be apparent, whether the child learns German or Chinese. All this would be part of the *phonetic* definition of the handicap. But when speakers have an intact auditory, articulatory and nervous system, it does not therefore follow that they will be able to learn the sound system of their language efficiently—and when there is a disability here (a 'specific' learning disability for some of the sounds of this system: see Chapter 3), each language has to be studied in its own terms. A child with an immature or deviant pronunciation of English will come across very differently from one with an immature or deviant pronunciation of French or Chinese. The assessment procedures will have to be different, and remedial work would proceed along quite different lines.

To say that a child has a 'poor pronunciation', then, does not help very much, until it is made clear whether we view his problem as being primarily a biological one (as conventionally defined in terms of anatomical, physiological or neurological abnormality), or as a psycholinguistic one (as conventionally defined in terms of the learning of psychological processes or linguistic rules). And, of course, many children suffer simultaneously from both kinds of handicap. Cleft palate children, for instance, will have a poor pronunciation which is explicable, to some extent, by their anatomical deficiency and the associated neurophysiological abnormalities. But other aspects of their pronunciation problem may not be so easily explicable, and suggest that there may be elements of a learning difficulty as part of the history of that handicap too. Part of the problem of making a good diagnosis and planning appropriate remedial help in this area, of course, is due to the complex way in which phonetic and phonological aspects of a disorder interact and overlap. It is especially easy to assume, in cases of severe physical handicap, that the problems are solely phonetic in character; but the existence of phonological learning problems in these children is widespread, and may be universal.

A similar process of reasoning applies to the study of written language. We may distinguish the range of marks which the human hand (with an implement) can produce and the human eye perceive, and the much more restricted range of marks which actually turn up in a language. The general study of human mark-making and mark-reception has no widely agreed name, but it is sometimes referred to as *graphetics*, on analogy with phonetics. The study of the mark system (more usually, the writing-system, or orthography) of a particular language is known as *graphology*. And, in a similar manner to the above discussion of sounds, we can distinguish between the biological factors which promote the development of an ability to read and write, and the psycholinguistic factors which impede it. To say that a child has 'poor reading', then, does not help much, until we have attempted to disentangle these two variables. One of the reasons why the term *dyslexia* is so confusing, of course, it that it leaves open whether the disorder is best viewed as essentially a neurological syndrome or a psycholinguistic one (see Chapter 3).

The range of linguistic variables discussed so far are to do with the relatively 'tangible' dimension of language structure—the strings of sounds, words and structures that come 'out of the mouth and into the ear', or 'out of the hand and into the eye'. The study of signing would have led to a similar structural account, though terminology would have differed to some extent. But if we turn now to the study of language in use, a quite different range of variables is implicated, as here we are dealing with the analysis of the *situations* in which language is found, and of the people who are involved in the act of communication. To impose some order on the enormous scope of this dimension, it is common to identify three broad parameters of variability, relating to temporal, social and psychological factors. First, *temporal* variation in language use refers to the way in which language changes over time, both in the long term (as when Anglo-Saxon develops into modern English) and in the short term (as in contemporary debates about English usage). Secondly, *social* variation in language use refers to the way in which language varies in terms of the regional or social background of the users, a domain which includes such notions as dialect, occupation, social status and social role, and which is generally studied under the heading of *sociolinguistics*. The socio-linguistic consequences of biological difference (such as sex, age, or handicap—'Does he take sugar?', as the title of a radio series about disabled people once put it) can also be included in this category. Thirdly, *psychological* variation in language use refers to the way in which language varies in terms of the capacities of the individual user, a domain which includes such notions as memory, attention, intelligence and personality, and which is generally studied under the heading of *psycholinguistics* (see Chapter 4). The study of individual differences, and of task effects on language, is also a major concern of the psycholinguist, as is the field of language learning, which is usually placed under this heading because of its dependence on cognitive abilities. The more restricted field of child language acquisition is therefore often referred to as *developmental* psycholinguistics.

The distinction between language structure and language use is a simple and attractive one, but it is misleading in one important respect. There are several features of language which cannot be identified without the equal participation of both dimensions. Terminology varies, but these days reference is generally made to them under the heading of *pragmatics*, and recently the pragmatic aspects of language development and language handicap have attracted particular attention (e.g. Ochs and Schieffelin 1979, Gallagher and Prutting 1983). Pragmatics has received many definitions, but essentially it refers to the study of the factors which govern users' choice of utterance, arising out of the social setting of which they are a part. It includes such matters as the assumptions which people make when they communicate, the intentions underlying what they say, the way context influences the amount they say or the way they say it, the turn-taking which makes a conversation run smoothly, the appropriateness of the subject-matter to a situation, and much more. Problems of a pragmatic kind are widespread in the study of language handicap, due to the limited awareness Ps may have of the nature of linguistic interaction, and the uncertainty many adults feel about how they should act when they encounter a handicapped person. Nor are professionals free of pragmatic uncertainty, and much of the current debate over what level of language to use to a child, whether we should speak or sign or do both, whether we should adopt a structured or a free conversational therapeutic style, and so on, illustrates the relevance of this topic to the work. Language handicap is first and foremost an interactive phenomenon: until we talk to Ps, we have no way of knowing whether they are linguistically handicapped or not. The implications of this axiom will be discussed in Chapter 5.

Recent textbooks on pragmatics (e.g. Leech 1983, Levinson 1983) illustrate the great breadth of the subject, and in their different approaches and emphases show how it is not yet possible to present a single classification of pragmatic variables which would satisfy everyone. At one extreme, pragmatics is closely related to semantics, and to other structural levels of language— so much so that some scholars would be prepared to call it a 'level' of language structure. At the other extreme, pragmatics is closely related to sociolinguistics and psycholinguistics, focusing upon matters of usage and extralinguistic context which have no direct relationship to language structure. In relation to the first extreme, there are clear cases where it is possible to make a pragmatic 'error' by wrongly using aspects of language structure—using *tu* instead of *vous* in certain circumstances in French, for example. On the other hand, it may also be a pragmatic 'error' if I tell a joke at a funeral, but here there is nothing in the structure of the English language which will explain what I have done wrong, and doubtless the same effect would be encountered in most other speech communities. Because of this range of subject-matter, it is in my view premature to talk of 'pragmatic disorders', as it is not possible to provide an unequivocal theoretical definition of what is involved. But the importance of pragmatic factors in the investigation of language handicap is undeniable.

These observations about language structure and use are sum-marized in Figure 2, which also shows the point of connection

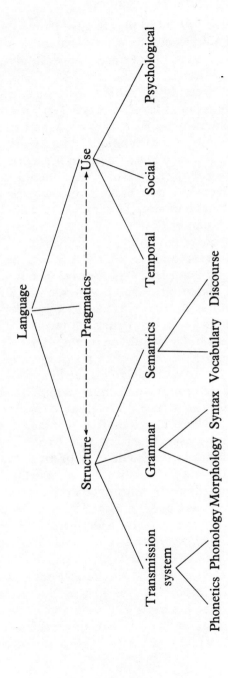

Figure 2 The main areas of spoken language structure and use

with Figure 1. The linguistic component of Figure 1 is represented by two main channels, or modes: the auditory-vocal channel,
and its visual encoding. Each channel divides immediately into
the main active and passive linguistic skills: listening/speaking
and reading/writing. And each skill is then analysed from the
viewpoints of structure and use. The model is a promising one.
The next step, accordingly, is to illustrate the way in which it can
be used as part of a clinical linguistic perspective, to elucidate
problems encountered in various fields of language handicap.

3

Two specific encounters

A good transcription and a theory of levels, taken together, constitute one of the most powerful tools available for the study of language handicap. The information they provide can act as the foundation for all subsequent reasoning about linguistic diagnosis, assessment and intervention. But they are of value long before these clinical goals are achieved, for they can contribute greatly to conceptual clarification, and help to determine research procedures and priorities. To illustrate this, I shall look at the kinds of problem which impede progress in clinical language studies, choosing two of the major handicapping conditions—aphasia in adults, and specific learning disability in children.

Aphasia

The importance of levels, and of linguistic hierarchy in general, has already been introduced with reference to the problems of aphasia classification (p.36). From a linguistic point of view, the central question is to determine the depth of detail at which useful descriptive statements should be made. At one extreme, there are the maximally general characterizations of the disorder which ignore levels altogether (such as 'fluent' versus 'non-fluent'). At the other extreme, there are the maximally detailed specifications of all the linguistic variables encountered in a sample, as presented in a set of profiles. Between, there are innumerable possibilities. Some scholars are satisfied with a classification of aphasic errors which recognizes only the three primary levels, with little or no subclassification: 'phonological' or 'phonemic' errors are seen alongside 'grammatical' or 'syntactic' errors, and 'semantic' or 'lexical' errors. We often have to 'see through' traditional clinical terminology to establish that a levels approach is in use; for example, the notion of *paraphasia* at first glance seems to be defined in a way which cuts across the various levels (e.g. 'the production of unintended syllables, words or phrases during the effort to speak' (Goodglass and Kaplan 1972: p.8), but the real use of this notion recognizes them, through its classification of *phonemic paraphasia* (phonological level), *verbal* and *neologistic paraphasias* (semantic level). Some classifications collapse into a single category notions which belong to different levels: for example, Ludlow (1981: Table 1) has as two of his categories 'impaired articulation and melody' (which seems to bring together an aspect of phonetics and one of phonology) and 'impaired fluency and syntax' (an aspect of phonetics/phonology plus an aspect of grammar). Others operate neatly with binary classifications within levels, probably the most well-known one being the distinction between *agrammatic* and *paragrammatic* speech within the level of grammar (though the involvement of semantic factors in this distinction must not be ignored). A classification in terms of levels of use is routinely made in aphasia tests, recognizing such distinctions as mode of communication (speaking, listening comprehension, reading, writing) and task (repetition, confrontation naming). Coltheart (1983: Chapter 18), in addressing the question of what counts as a useful descriptive level at which to work, considers the following specifications (among others) to be helpful: 'using function words in spon- taneous speech', 'speech comprehension at the single-sentence level' and 'reading comprehension at the paragraph level'.

However, when we consider the properties of an 'ideal' aphasia theory, it is plain that the depth of descriptive detail presented by these approaches is still a long way from what is required. A theory of aphasia ought to be predictive, in the sense that from a precise specification of neurological damage, it should be possible to derive predictions concerning P's linguistic behaviour at any point in time during the recovery process. Such a theory would also have to take into account the facilitating or hindering effects of formal interventions, in the course of therapy or rehabilitation. Now, despite the limited progress which has been made in this direction, everyday clinical work has no alternative but to proceed as if the theory existed. Ts will make assumptions to guide their therapy, on the basis of the medical case history and accompanying general observation; and their intention will be to change P's behaviour in a controlled manner, through the use of treatment hypotheses deriving from an ongoing analysis of their own stimuli and P's response. I see no point in an aphasia theory which is unable to make predictions about therapy. And it is in relation to therapy that the descriptive detail of the classifications referred to above proves to be inadequate.

For, how would Ts be able to interpret such notions as 'paraphasia' and 'word-finding problem', in order to carry out treatment? Even the more detailed specifications suggested by Coltheart are too general, in this respect: a much more precise statement about such notions as 'function word', 'non-verbal behaviour' or 'single sentence' is required, before Ts could devise a treatment programme based on this rationale. Which function words are strong, which weak, and in which contexts? Which features of non-verbal behaviour are strong, which weak, and related to which aspects of conversation? Which kinds of single sentence? Which kinds of paragraph? Ts have to begin a session of treatment with a specific interaction, using specific sentences of a particular type, and they must monitor P's response, which also uses specific sentences (whether normal or abnormal) of a particular type. The treatment session does not deal with 'function words': it deals with a particular function word, or set of words, in conditions that ought to be carefully specified. The goal is to establish the use of one or other of these words in P's behaviour. And it is by no means uncommon for whole sections of a session to be devoted to the eliciting and training of a single item. An assessment made at the beginning and end of such a training period has therefore to be sufficiently detailed to capture the progress which may have been made, in order to inform further decisions as to how the next stage in therapy might proceed. At this level of concern, the task of description is inevitably an extremely detailed one, and the gap between it and the level of generality illustrated above is enormous.

But it is not solely aphasia therapy which is undermined by the lack of appropriately detailed descriptions. It can also be argued that theoretical research into aphasia is being hindered by a reluctance to look beneath the general labels and to provide a more precise specification of the disorder. The point can be illustrated from one of the most frequently cited diagnostic criteria, *agrammatism*, which is often used as if it were a well-defined notion, but which on examination turns out not to be the case. The imprecision hinges on the 'amount' of grammar which is permitted to be subsumed under the term. At one extreme, it would seem that the term refers to the whole of the grammatical level, as in the definition of Critchley (1970: p.16): 'an aphasic disorder which impairs syntax rather than vocabulary'. Most of grammar is implicated in Jakobson's account of agrammatism as a contiguity disorder:

> The syntactical rules organizing words into higher units are lost, [and this] causes the degeneration of the sentence into a mere 'word heap' . . . Word order becomes chaotic; the ties of grammatical coordination and subordination . . . are dissolved . . . words endowed with purely grammatical functions, like conjunctions, prepositions, pronouns, and articles, disappear first . . . and a typical feature . . . is the abolition of inflection. (1954/71: pp.251-2)

At the other extreme, agrammatism is used to refer to just one aspect of grammatical analysis—the factor of so-called 'grammatical' or 'function' words (another example of the bias introduced by the Indo-European languages, incidentally (cf. p.38), for there are many languages to which this concept does not readily apply). For example, Eisenson says:

> Typically, agrammatism is characterised by the patient's errors or omissions in the use of functional words . . . which serve to establish contextual relationships (grammatical context) of spoken and written content. (1973: p.20)

Albert *et al.* (1981: p.30) describe it as 'a near total absence of the "small grammatical words" of the language'. Some definitions stress the morphological aspect of the problem, by drawing attention to the loss of inflections (e.g. Albert *et al.* 1981); others ignore morphology, and give a definition solely in terms of syntax (e.g. Nicolosi, Harryman and Kresheck's definition as 'impairment of the ability to produce words in their correct sequence', a definition they have based on Wood, in Travis (1963)). Albert *et al.* begin with morphology, but end up with an account which implicates the whole of the system of grammatical relationships:

> Closer inspection of agrammatic speech suggests that this style has a more complex explanation than a mere dropping out of grammatical elements. In fact there appears to be a basic loss of the concept of words as having a functional role in a sentence. The severe agrammatic uses words as disconnected, nominalized ideas, which can be placed contiguously without any expressed grammatical connection between them. (1981: p.30)

Several problems present themselves, as we try to make sense of such a range of definitions. To take the statement of Albert *et al.*: to what extent is this last characterization a matter of 'agrammatic speech' in general, or, as they say, 'severe' agrammatic speech in particular? And would they wish to maintain that, from the observation that there is no 'expressed' grammatical connection, there is no underlying grammatical connection made at all? Or, to take Eisenson's statement: 'In severe form, agrammatism may be expressed as *telegrammatism*. All functional words and grammatical markers may be omitted' (1973: p.21). The *all* seems to be the point at issue, for he gives as a 'more typical' example of agrammatic production the sentence *I eggs and eat and drink coffee*. But if this is typical, how does it square with the various accounts which mention the omission of pronouns and conjunctions in agrammatism? In fact, there is considerable uncertainty as to the function words which are omitted in agrammatic speech. Albert *et al.* list them as 'the customary articles, pronouns, noun and verb inflections [*sic*], auxiliaries' (p.30); Goodglass (1976:

p.237) says 'articles, connective words, auxiliaries and inflections'; Eisenson (p.20) says 'articles, prepositions and conjunctions'; Robbins (1951) says 'auxiliaries and relational words' in one definition, 'conjunctions and other subordinate [*sic*] words' in another, and adds that 'words are uttered in incorrect sequence, infinitives are misused'.

Rough characterizations of this kind may be generally satisfactory for impressionistic clinical purposes, but as soon as a more rigorous approach is required, a clearer and more comprehensive description comes to be essential. Research studies in neurolinguistics and neuropsychology, for example, cannot afford to be loose in their handling of the notion of agrammatism, especially when statistical studies are involved, or in case studies where the meticulous analysis of lists of examples and counterexamples is routine. And yet, the looseness is universal. In a valuable review of deep dyslexia, for example, Coltheart asks whether such Ps are agrammatic, points out that several of those studied in his paper were not, and concludes that 'agrammatism of speech is *not* one of the symptoms of deep dyslexia' (1980: pp.35-7). A little later in the same volume, Morton begins his paper with the words: 'In spite of their trouble with reading, their agrammatism and nonfluency', referring to his group of Ps (1980: p.189), and Saffran *et al.*, in the same volume (1980: p.382) state that 'Almost all of the patients would be classified as agrammatic.' But what are the descriptive criteria used in this debate? Coltheart defines agrammatism thus: 'function words and inflections are selectively absent from speech which is still relatively meaningful and communicative' (*ibid.*: p.35); Saffran *et al.* say that it 'consists mostly of concrete nouns . . . contains relatively few verb forms . . . and is notably lacking in functors' (*ibid.*: p.382). Whatever the reality of the situation, it is plain that with overlapping definitions of this kind, points of similarity and difference may be being obscured. Unless everyone uses precisely the same set of descriptive criteria, comparisons can be weakened to the point of vacuity.

What must be appreciated is that there is no 'correct' definition of a notion such as 'function word', and it is certainly not possible to take it as self-evident. The distinction between 'content words' and 'function words' (or whatever terminology is used) is not clear-cut, as has long been recognized in the linguistics literature (see, for example, the special volume of *Lingua* (1967) devoted to the topic of word-classes). Function words are said to be empty of meaning, to have solely grammatical function. In fact, hardly any of the words considered functional have no referential meaning (the clearest cases are the infinitival particle *to*, and the 'empty' uses of *there* and *it* in *there's a horse in the street* and *it was yesterday I saw him*). Most function words have some kind of referential meaning (all the prepositional or pronominal items, for example), and some lists of such words contain many items whose supposed grammatical status is open to question. In the deep dyslexia volume referred to above (Coltheart, Patterson and Marshall 1980), for instance, there is an appendix listing function word paralexias used by certain Ps. They include items such as *had, was, to, the, not, or, am* and *are*; but they also include *on, down, most, while, where, just, neither, both* and *almost*, which seem to be semantically at a remove from the first set; and also *perhaps, sometimes, something, ever, generally, instead, never, seldom, therefore, usually* and *several*, which are really somewhat unexpected. After all, if such items are included, where do we draw the line between function and content word? If *sometimes* and *seldom* are included, why not *often, frequently, regularly*, and thousands more of the adverbials available in English (see Quirk, Greenbaum, Leech and Svartvik forthcoming: Chapter 8)? A line may have to be drawn, to enable research to proceed, but in our present state of knowledge of the areas of grammar involved, it is going to be an arbitrary one. It certainly cannot be left to take care of itself.

Nor is agrammatism an isolated example. A concept such as 'word-finding' is likewise implicated, in view of the way in which this notion may be made to depend on a word classification principle similar to the one above. Albert *et al.*, for example, see word-finding as 'an estimate of the balance between contentive words and grammatical filler words', contentive words being 'nouns, principal verbs, adjectives and adverbs' (1981: p.31). They would presumably class *sometimes, usually*, etc. as content words, compared with the approach cited in the previous paragraph. But most discussion of word-finding problems is not even so specific, most authors apparently seeing the concept of

'word-finding' as so self-evident that it does not require definition. Yet we have only to ask 'What is it that is to be found?' to see
that the term hides a nest of methodological and theoretical
problems. At one extreme, *all* the words in a language can be said
to present difficulties of retrieval, including all classes of 'content'
words and all the 'grammatical' words containing some degree of
specifiable meaning. At the other extreme, only one sub-class of
'content' words is considered to be relevant, as when word-
finding difficulties are cited only as part of the discussion of
anomia (as in the index to Eisenson (1973), for example). In some
contexts, it would seem to be the word in a specific grammatical
and phonological form which has to be found (*take, takes, took,
taken, taking*). In other contexts, a more abstract sense of 'word' is
clearly intended—the 'underlying form' of the various grammatical and phonological possibilities (the *lexical item* or *lexeme* TAKE).
A lexeme is the minimal unit of meaning in the semantic system of
a language (see Lyons 1977: Chapter 1), and the notion has
proved valuable in enabling the semantic analysis of vocabulary to
proceed independently of the complications introduced by the
constraints of grammatical form. But its potential as a means of
refining and making precise the concept of 'word-finding problem' has yet to be appreciated.

We can see this if we look at just some of the possibilities that
the notion of 'word-finding' can subsume. A particular form of a
lexeme may be lost, such as the noun *switch* as opposed to the verb
switch, or the 3rd person form of the verb (*switches*), or the first
part of a (multi-word) lexeme (saying *on* for *switch on*, for
instance). Or the whole of a lexeme may be 'lost', as when all
forms of the lexeme, regardless of context, are unusable (*switch,
switches, switching, switch on*, etc.). Or again, a particular use of a
lexeme may be lost (*switch* in the sense of 'electric switch', but not
in the sense of 'change direction'), or a particular relationship
between one lexeme and another (oppositeness, for example—
switch on versus *switch off*, *big* versus *small*). The study of the way
in which the lexemes of a language are organized into *semantic
fields*, and are linked by specific *semantic* (or *sense*) *relations*, such
as synonymy, oppositeness and hyponymy (the relationship of
inclusion), constitutes one of the major themes of contemporary

semantics, but it is an approach which has not been systematically applied to the analysis of aphasia (see further, Crystal 1981: Chapter 5).

Aphasia tests often inquire after particular synonyms or antonyms, of course, but the tasks are always somewhat artificial, and do not take into account the range of contextual factors which constitute the real difficulty in handling a language's vocabulary. As an example of the 'decontextualised' approach, we might consider the kind of question put to Ps, in which they are asked (in so many words) for the opposite of, say, *run*. An inadequate response may well be due to the fact that there is no single, 'correct' opposite for this lexeme: *run* has several opposites, depending on the context in which it is used, as the following examples illustrate:

> It's not enough to run round the track; you have to *jump* the hurdles as well.
> I *walked* towards the bus-stop; but when I saw the bus coming I started to run.
> The engine was running nicely, but then there was a sharp noise and it *stopped.*
> My horse isn't running; it's been *scratched*.
> The buses aren't running; they're *on strike*.
> The play's not running any more; it's been *taken off*.

Most lexemes in the language have many such 'opposites', and the commonest have most of all. Without adequate contextual awareness, then, it is not possible to make sense of P's responses. Ts may present a task in which they assume that the opposite of *run* is *walk*; Ps however may respond by saying *scratch*, which might easily be interpreted either as a comprehension difficulty with *run*, or a word-finding problem with *walk*, or both, unless we thought to check the horse-racing context. And similar problems arise when we consider the way in which Ps might be using synonyms, or any other sense relation. The only solution, of course, is to ensure that Ts' approach to lexical assessment and remediation is given an adequate descriptive foundation: they must be aware, in principle, of the range and complexity of the semantic factors involved, and have available, as a matter of routine, a systematic description of the lexical possibilities being drawn upon by Ps. Primitive lexical descriptions, more than adequate for basic clinical needs, already exist: they are called dictionaries and thesauri, or subtle combinations of these genres, as found in the Longman *Lexicon*, which is an immensely valuable reference book for clinical work. But are these books ever seen as being essential pieces of clinical equipment? And are they ever routinely consulted as a preliminary to condemning P's lexical response as 'random', or to constructing a lexical teaching programme?

The cases of agrammatism and word-finding are only two of the notions which have received inadequate description in terms of the main linguistic levels and their sub-divisions. Agrammatism is primarily a grammatical notion, but it has been only partially explicated in its reliance on function words and morphological structure; it now needs to be investigated using a more abstract set of syntactic relations within the frame of reference of a reasonably comprehensive descriptive model—for example, such relations as subject, object, complement and verb, used in association with the clause, phrase and other aspects of grammatical hierarchy (see Crystal 1981: Chapter 4). Word-finding is primarily a semantic notion, but it too has been only partially explicated, in terms of simple quantitative notions such as word frequency, word length and word association norms (Lesser 1978: pp.107ff.); it now needs to be investigated using a set of qualitative semantic relations, both syntagmatic and paradigmatic, so that lexical assessment and treatment can be seen within the frame of reference of an emerging system of structured semantic fields. But the descriptive refinement of already available aphasiological notions is only the tip of the iceberg of linguistic enquiry into the disorder, using the model of levels. There remain wholly uncharted areas of aphasic behaviour, areas which are undoubtedly central to our understanding and treatment of the condition, but which have received little or no study because of the limited account which has been taken of theoretical linguistic insights in clinical training and practice. The point can be briefly illustrated from each of the main linguistic levels.

From the point of view of grammar and semantics, apart from

the issues already noted, there is a considerable neglect of the hierarchical properties of sentence construction, especially the relationships between sentence and clause, and between clause and phrase (phrase and word, and word and morpheme, as we have seen, are routinely investigated). To illustrate the problem, firstly at the grammatical level, we may take the following sentence sequence:

You.
You asked.
You asked John.
You asked my brother.

Each sentence increases by one word, but there is a qualitatively different jump which takes place between the third and the fourth sentences. The fourth sentence is not simply a linear string of four separate words: the relationship between *my* and *brother* is closer than that between *my* and *asked*, or *my* and *you*. This is conventionally illustrated in the form of a constituency diagram, such as:

you   asked   my   brother

(though this is only one way of representing the structural relationships involved). However we calculate the 'processing load' involved in these sentences, it should be evident that the jump from the third to the fourth sentence involves two extra factors—the extra word, and the extra level of sentence structure. It would not therefore follow that, because Ps could handle some four-word sentences (such as *I saw John today*, where there is no hierarchical structure), they would be able to handle this one. They may be able to say (or comprehend) *you asked John* and *my brother*, as separate utterances, but the conflating of the two might be beyond them. Moreover, it does not follow that, because Ps can handle hierarchy after the verb (as in *You asked my brother*), they can handle it before the verb (as in *My brother asked me*); indeed, differential ability in this respect is the norm, for both adults and children (cf. Quirk *et al.* forthcoming: Chapter 17; Crystal, Fletcher and Garman 1976: p.114). And the possibility of interference from other grammatical and semantic factors must be considered (in statement versus question, positive versus negative construction, using animate versus inanimate nouns, following static versus dynamic verbs (e.g. *see* versus *hit*), and so on), as well as phonological factors (such as placement of nuclear tone). Whether we are studying comprehension or production, the relationship between clause and phrase elements always needs to be taken systematically into acount. And a similar set of factors needs to be borne in mind when we look at more complex clauses, and the sequencing of clauses within sentences (see further, Chapter 4).

In recent years, some progress has been made in the analysis of aphasic speech using the concept of grammatical hierarchy, but the potentially more fruitful corresponding analysis in semantic terms has not been invoked. The distinction between grammar and semantics here is best illustrated with a sentence, analysed from both points of view:

	John	kicked	the ball
Grammar	Subject	Verb	Object
Semantics	Actor	Action	Goal

That the two levels are not the same notions masquerading under different labels can be shown by using other sentences:

	The ball	was kicked	by John
Grammar	Subject	Verb	Adverbial
Semantics	Goal	Action	Actor

In the first sentence, the Subject is the semantic Actor; in the second it is the semantic Goal of the Action. The clauses and clause elements of grammar play a number of semantic 'roles', which have been variously labelled by different scholars, and this constitutes an illuminating avenue of enquiry into the nature of aphasic disability. This is especially the case in relation to the more 'fluent' speech characteristic of Wernicke's aphasia, where a grammatical analysis is often unilluminating, as a wide range of sentence patterns is in use. Such speech is often said to be semantically 'empty', 'low in information', containing 'unnecessary words', 'circumlocutions' and various kinds of 'jargon'. On the other hand, there seems to have been little attempt to provide a qualitative analysis of these notions—to describe the kinds of circumlocution, to see whether certain semantic elements are more prone to circumlocution, and so on. Nor does anyone seem to have investigated these issues in relation to the semantic load carried by T's verbal stimulus to P (though for some programmatic suggestions, see Crystal 1981: Chapter 5).

Yet surely this kind of information is basic to our understanding of the condition? Faced with a question such as *What is a key?*, Ps may respond by keeping their meaning mainly constant, and varying their grammar (*A key opens a door, A door is opened by a key, It's a key to open a door*, etc.); or by keeping the grammar mainly constant, and varying the semantic content (*I open a door, You open cupboards, You lock a door*;); or of course by some combination. Similarly, Ts may vary the grammatical ways in which they ask the same question (*What can you do with a key?*, *What's a key for?*, etc.); or vary the meaning while maintaining the same grammatical form (*Do you eat things with it?, Do you open things with it?*, etc.); or of course vary both factors at once. Ps may be unable to process certain semantic elements, yet have a facility in coping with others; for example, they might be unable to handle lexemes when these have an Actor role to play in a sentence, but be able to handle them when they function as Goal (*cat bite* versus *bite cat*). They may have a preference for certain semantic roles, tending to focus on these first, to the neglect of other elements in the sentence— something which may happen as part of comprehension or production. For example, one P focused on any element which had a temporal role to play: in answer to a question such as *Where did you go yesterday?*, he would focus on *yesterday* and talk about when it was, which day it was, and so on; in his own spontaneous speech, he would tend to begin a sentence with a temporal expression and use such expressions repeatedly in his speech (*well sometimes/ I like to quite often really/—on Sundays/ I go you see/ often/. . .*). Rather than discount this kind of monologue as 'empty', 'stereotyped' or 'automatic', it makes more sense to investigate it systematically, and arrive at a description of the semantic roles and patterns which are being used, and which avoided. Only in this way can a norm be established for P, which can act as a baseline for subsequent evaluation of his linguistic progress.

The segmental (vowel, consonant, syllable) aspect of phonology is a familiar area in aphasiology, but even here there are glaring gaps. To begin with, there is a marked bias towards the study of consonant errors, often to the exclusion of vowels. This is presumably a consequence of the tradition in articulation testing, where for many years consonants were the only phenomena to be investigated; but it cannot be justified in relation to aphasia, where errors of vowel length and quality are common. And while consonant errors do tend to be in the majority, it must not be forgotten that vowel values can play an essential part in the distinguishing of pairs of consonants—final [p] and [b], for instance, are primarily distinguished in terms of the length of the preceding vowel, as in *cap/cab*, etc. Secondly, there has been little sign of the importance of taking into account a sound's distribution (cf. p.78) in relation to larger linguistic units, such as syllable, word, tone unit or phrase. There is still a marked tendency to talk about sounds globally—P's 'difficulty with [l]', for example, instead of his 'difficulty with [l] in word-initial position'. And indeed, despite all the use made of the term *phoneme*, there is still a predominance in the aphasia literature to think of phonemes as sounds, as physical entities, instead of what they are—abstract classes of sounds, contrasting units within a sound system.

The almost universal focus on the phoneme as the key to the understanding of aphasic phonology is clear from a review such as Lesser's (1978: Chapter 8), but this is by no means a satisfactory state of affairs. There are many other ways of studying phonological systems, and while some attention has been paid to the use of one of these (the distinctive feature frame of reference used in generative phonology), there are further approaches of considerable relevance to the analysis of aphasic errors, whose application has hardly begun. For example, we might examine those phonological processes which extend beyond the individual phoneme, and which apply to whole syllables, words or larger units (which have been variously referred to as 'prosodies' (Firth 1948) or 'phonological processes' (as in Ingram 1976)). The idea that a single process can explain the selection of certain sounds made by a speaker at different points in an utterance has proved to be helpful in studies of normal language acquisition and of child language disability (Grunwell 1981), and it seems likely that it would also be illuminating in the study of adult disorders. Several aphasiological notions seem tailor-made for analysis in terms of processes (for example, 'perseveration'), and the approach might help to resolve some of the puzzles left by previous characterizations of disorders. Conventional accounts of apraxia, for example, refer to inconsistency of phonological errors (cf. Lesser 1978: p.159). But is there really inconsistency, or is this the result of using only a phonemic model to investigate the disorder? Faced with a set of data where an item such as *pig* is recorded as [pig], [kig] and [sig], there seems to be inconsistency; but widening the scope of the enquiry may lead to explanations for the alternative forms. The /p/ may be realized as [k] under the influence of a following /k/, for example, as in *the pig is coming* (what is often referred to as an instance of 'consonant harmony'); the [s] may be the consequence of a preceding phoneme, as in *I see a pig*. We are not at the stage where it is possible to predict classes of error, or define the constraints on such processes as harmony; but there is a great deal to be gained by making use of the notion of process in analysing aphasic speech samples.

Lastly, within phonology, there is the neglect of non-segmental characteristics of language, especially of intonation, which has already been pointed out in relation to the need for transcriptional accuracy (p.42). In the absence of non-segmental transcriptions, there will obviously be little precise study of the way in which Ps control the forms and functions of intonation, stress, tempo, rhythm or pause, in relation to the rest of their language, and to the kinds of task they are called upon to perform. Equally, the way in which Ts make use of non-segmental variation in order to organize their stimuli, or to highlight a particular feature of language, has received little description (but see Crystal forthcoming). Recommendations about interaction remain controversial (for example, whether we should increase or decrease our tempo of speech stimuli to facilitate P's response), and diagnostic characterizations remain vague (for example, using general impressions about 'melody' or 'colour' of speech, and relying on a notion of 'dysprosody' whose phonetic or phonological status it is never possible to determine (see further, Crystal 1981: Chapter

3)). But the potential of this area for extending our understanding of aphasic symptomatology is enormous—in my view, more than in any other domain of clinical linguistic application.

Specific learning disability

I pick up the term 'specific learning disability' (or any of its near equivalents, such as 'specific learning problems') somewhat gingerly, for I have mixed feelings about it. On the one hand, I applaud the focus on learning, as an end in itself, and the associated focus on disability. On the other hand, I can make no sense of the term 'specific', and consider that its uncritical use obscures rather than clarifies the nature of the disabilities which we wish to understand. The reason for these mixed feelings will become clear if we look briefly at the history of the notion.

It is not difficult to see why the term was originally felt to be useful. People wished to draw a contrast with disabilities of a more global kind, in which there was fundamental brain damage, or other comparably general disturbances. A widely quoted definition illustrates this perspective (National Advisory Committee 1968):

Children with special [= specific] learning disabilities exhibit a disorder in one or more of the basic psychological processes involved in understanding or in using spoken or written language. These may be manifested in disorders of listening, thinking, talking, reading, writing, spelling, or arithmetic. They include conditions which have been referred to as perceptual handicaps, brain injury, minimal brain dysfunction, dyslexia, developmental aphasia, etc. They do not include learning problems which are primarily due to visual, hearing or motor handicaps, to mental retardation, emotional disturbance, or to environmental disadvantage.

The emphasis of this definition is fairly universal (cf. Tarnopol and Tarnopol 1976, Gearhart 1981), even though it raises several problems (such as the uncertain boundary between peripheral and central sensory handicap, or between minimal and severe brain damage), and even though practice varies greatly (for example, over whether we rigorously exclude all motor handicaps, and all environmental—presumably including all cultural—disadvantage). The point of the definition is to suggest that there is a significant discrepancy between a child's actual level of psycholinguistic functioning and the level of functioning we would expect, given normal intelligence and sensory capability. From this point of view, I suppose it was a natural enough move to use the term 'special' or 'specific' to refer to the more narrowly defined syndrome.

The trouble comes when we attempt to interpret the term in a positive way, and to operationalize the definition in order to get on with a clinical or educational job, such as assessment or remediation. It is then that we realize how unspecific the term 'specific' is. For what is specific about the disability characterized by the above definition? Is an 'imperfect ability to think' specific? Or an 'imperfect ability to speak'? Could we conceive of any *more general* psycholinguistic disabilities than those referred to in the definition? There is something odd about the use of the word 'specific' in this context. My dictionary gives one set of meanings for the word as 'precise, definite, explicit', and this the above definition is not, as is indicated by 'one or more' processes, and the overlaps already noted. The dictionary also gives a medical sense of the word, 'produced by a particular micro-organism (or the medicine that has a particular curative influence on a disease)', and I suspect many people attribute medical connotations to 'specific' when they encounter it. But in the absence of any neurological (or neuropsychological) aetiology for the condition, in our present state of knowledge, we cannot permit this interpretation. No-one should be fooled by the phrase 'basic psychological processes', as indicating a specific cause, for we do not know what these processes might be. Psychological theories compete for our attention in providing us with an account of them, but here there is much speculation and little orthodoxy. Terms like 'memory', 'perception' and 'attention' are widely used, and several operational tests are available to probe these notions; but the relationships which obtain between them, and between them and language, and how these relationships might be invoked when language learning breaks down—here no clear understanding exists.

Nor can the term be saved by an appeal to the learning categories excluded by the definition, as would be standard procedure when working with the notion of diagnosis by exclusion in medicine. In the medical model, one can make such a diagnosis only when the symptomatology for each disease is unambiguous, and thus the set of differentiating signs and symptoms clearly understood. In the field of learning disability, by contrast, these conditions do not obtain. We do not know what are the defining linguistic characteristics of emotional disturbance, mental retardation, hearing loss, or whatever, when these categories are presented to us in such a general way. Each of these fields is a research area in its own right, where it is now well known that any linguistic characterization is going to be extremely complex. Even in the most profoundly handicapped groups (such as severe mental retardation, or profound deafness), individual differences in linguistic skills abound, as is routinely recognized every day in classroom and clinic. And it is not at all clear whether the deficiencies in language manifested by, say, profoundly deaf people, are a result of their deafness, or of one of the other factors mentioned above (such as environmental disadvantage, or an inadequate educational method). So, when someone presents with a set of linguistic symptoms, it becomes a major analytical task to decide which symptoms relate to which causative factors. It is usually not possible to decide with any certainty, and the possibility of a specific learning disability existing *alongside* the more obvious factors can certainly never be ruled out. If deaf people have problems in learning to read, are these due to their deafness, or to a specific learning disability which coexists with their deafness? It is difficult if not impossible to answer such questions, and as a result the term 'specific' cannot be saved by appeal to a process of diagnosis by exclusion. On the contrary, all that is left when we attempt to eliminate these other factors is something very unspecific indeed: it would have been better to call the syndrome 'unspecific learning disability'.

Now I am not merely making a terminological point, in all of this, as in Chapter 1. My concern is with the real-world implications of this argument for anyone working in the field of linguistic diagnosis, assessment or intervention. I wish to argue that to apply the label 'specific learning disability' to a child is not the end of the diagnostic process, as many people assume: it is only the beginning. And I wish to argue, also, that this notion, as currently defined, cannot be an acceptable foundation for clinical or educational work, without massive refinement. The problem we all have to face is how to refine the notion, to make it useful to teacher and clinician alike—in a word, how do we make the notion of 'specific' specific?

This is where the levels model of language comes in. We need to work with a theoretical apparatus which at one extreme is sufficiently general to map into the categories used in general definitions of 'specific learning disability', and at the other extreme is sufficiently detailed to identify the precise targets of daily teaching and therapy. At one extreme: notions such as 'reading', 'speaking', etc. At the other extreme: problems such as children who read *saw* as *was*, or who are having trouble with consonant clusters such as [pl] and [bl] in their speech. The unfortunate thing is that few theoreticians have opportunity (or sometimes motivation) to study classroom and clinic interaction in relation to their models (which is, I think, largely due to a bias towards experimental studies in the relevant branches of psychology); and few Ts have opportunity (or sometimes motivation) to step back from their daily preoccupations and attempt to describe and evaluate what they are doing. In clinical linguistics, I see a possible bridge between these two extremes: the bias towards routine observation, description and analysis of T-P interaction leads to the development of diagnostic and remedial hypotheses, and these in turn motivate specific courses of action (see p.32, and Chapter 5). What is not possible, in our present state of knowledge, is to make anything other than the vaguest generalizations about *groups* of children, and therefore it is not really diagnosis in the usual sense. Each child is unique in several respects; each is reminiscent of certain other children, but is the same as none of them. It is always the way, at present: the individual differences stand out, at the expense of the common features. We can see the trees, but not the wood. Indeed, at present we are only at the stage of realizing that there *is* a wood. And it will be years before the main pathways are traced through it.

To illustrate the way bridges can be built, let us apply the hierarchy of levels represented in Figures 1 and 2 (pp.47,56), and follow one of the possible paths down it. The vaguest possible characterization of P's language handicap would be to use the categories given at the top of the figure—to say, for example, that they have an 'auditory-vocal' language handicap. This leaves unclear whether speaking or listening is involved, or both. Let us assume that the handicap affects spoken language only. The next step presents us with the possibility that the handicap may be either in the structure of the spoken language, or in its use, or again, in both. Let us assume that only structure is involved. The next step asks us to locate the handicap at one of the levels of semantics, grammar or transmission system, or in terms of some combination of these. Let us assume that the transmission system is the only level affected. We now have to determine whether the handicap is phonetic or phonological in type, or both. Let us assume that it is phonological.

We have reached the bottom of Figure 2, but there is still some way to go before we arrive at an analysis which is capable of being introduced directly into the classroom or clinic. To say that P has a 'phonological' handicap is, indeed, a relatively specific description—at least, compared with those used higher up the figure— but it is still somewhat abstract. Each of the structural headings needs to be broken down further. Within phonology, the next step would be to make a distinction between those features of sound which can be identified as segments, and those which cannot. Under the first heading, we have various consonants and vowels, and the ways these combine to form syllables. Under the second heading, we have the prosodic and paralinguistic effects, of the kind outlined in Chapter 2—effects which stretch over whole words, sentences and even at times longer units of speech. P's phonological handicap may be segmental, or non-segmental, or both. Let us assume it is segmental. The next step is to recognize formally the distinction just alluded to: P's handicap may be the result of difficulties with consonants, or with vowels, or both. Let us assume consonants are the main problem. The next step, accordingly, is to distinguish the different kinds of consonants, using the standard criteria—place of articulation, manner of articulation, voicing, and so on. Let us assume that P's handicap is basically a matter of place of articulation. The next step is to identify particular segments within the category of place— bilabial, dental, velar, and so on—which correlate with the symbols provided by a system of phonetic transcription. Let us assume that velar consonants are the ones mainly affected. At this point, therefore, we can identify particular sounds, and transcribe them using the range of symbols available (cf. p.45).

Here, many people would think it was time to stop, for how could there be anything more detailed than the identification of a specific sound, such as [k]? But in fact there are two further steps to take into account, which move us back in the direction of grammar and semantics. We have to ask the grammatical question: where is the sound [k] being used? In what part of a word— at the beginning, in the middle, or at the end? Sometimes, even, in what part of a sentence? The sound's *distribution* is an important dimension of its description. If Ps have trouble with velars only at the ends of words, their problem is rather different from Ps who have velar trouble in initial position as well. And lastly, we have to ask the semantic (lexical) question: where is the sound [k] being used, in the sense of what *kind* of word? Is it only used in the words *cat* or *car*, or in a wider range of words?

This whole chain of reasoning is illustrated in Figure 3. Now, and only now, once we have reached the bottom level of the hierarchy, are we in the world of the classroom or clinic. At this level, we are dealing with Ps who make errors in individual sounds in individual words, such as replacing [k] by [t] in *cat* or *car*. To work on this problem, a speech therapist would have to choose specific words in specific sentences, and work out specific contrasts for P to practise, using specific materials. Likewise, if a teacher were to trace the argument to its conclusion, but in the context of the teaching of reading. Everyone notices the child who reads *was* as *saw*, or vice versa. This again is a quite specific confusion, concerning certain types of words which are reverse images of each other; and if Ts chose to work on this confusion, they would have to choose specific words in specific sentences, and work out specific contrasts for P to practise, using specific materials.

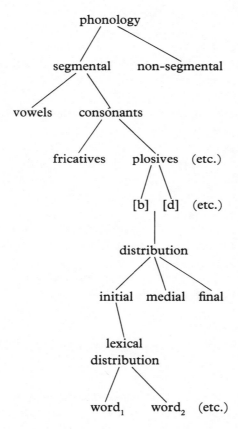

Figure 3   A possible decision hierarchy within phonology

At any given point in a teaching day, or therapy session, T is working on specific problems of this kind—and obviously the more systematically we can identify the range of these problems, and organize our approach to them, the better. But listing a range of problems does not constitute a diagnosis, for which some degree of generalization needs to be made. The hierarchy in

Figures 1-3 allows several degrees of generalization, and there-fore—and this is the important point—several *levels* of diagnosis. It would be perfectly proper (though admittedly somewhat unusual) to refer to P's handicap in any of the following terms, as we move upwards through the figures:

> P has a disability in final velar production—that is, trouble in using velar consonants in final position in words in speech, but no problem in perceiving these sounds in the same position in listening;
> P has a disability in velar production—that is, any velar, anywhere in the word;
> P has a disability in final consonant production—what is sometimes referred to as an 'open syllable' problem;
> P has a disability in consonant production—that is, all consonants are affected, his speech consisting of little more than vowels;
> P has a disability in the production of sound segments—neither vowels nor consonants are clear, but prosody is unaffected;
> P has a disability in phonology—both the segmental and the non-segmental aspects are affected;
> P has a disability in phonology and grammar, but only in production;
> P has a disability in phonology and grammar, but in compre-hension as well as production;

and so we might continue, incorporating semantics, language use, and other modes of communication, and allowing for different combinations of sub-sets of difficulties under each heading. The number of possible symptom-complexes, when all these variables are taken into account, is as near infinite as makes no difference, for real cases are not as simple as the hypothetical ones just listed. There are, for instance, over a quarter of a million substitution patterns within the plosive consonant system alone! The aim of research is therefore to determine the dependencies between these categories, in order to reduce the set of disability patterns to manageable proportions. And this is where a great deal of progress is currently being made, in identifying putative linguistic syndromes, made up of clusters of phonological, grammatical and semantic features, viewed in relation to the relevant variables of language in use (which will account for P's differential performance as he encounters different tasks, Ts, settings, and so on). For those involved in the work, it is a long-term programme indeed, but a programme from which several useful insights have already emerged (some of which will be discussed further in Chapter 4).

In the context of the present chapter, it will be apparent that the conception of 'specific learning disability' as a hierarchy of levels of linguistic difficulty is itself an important insight, in that it helps to impose some order on the chaos of observations which are made in relation to that heading. But this conception carries with it certain other implications about the *integrated* nature of language disabilities—a specific problem in one area being seen in the light of the strengths and weaknesses of other areas. As already suggested, the list of 'disabilities' given above is unreal— not least because it is very rarely the case that single modes of language are affected. Problems of writing usually mean problems of reading; problems of speaking usually mean problems of listening; and, the most important of all, in view of recent research, problems of reading usually mean problems of speaking and listening. The interdependency of the four main language modes is widely recognized these days (especially, in the UK, since the Bullock Report's (1975) emphasis upon the point). The teaching of reading is seen within the context of children's previous linguistic experience—that is, their speaking and listening experience. The usual criticism of traditional reading schemes was how far away they were from the kind of language children were familiar with (cf. Crystal 1976: Chapter 3), and more recent schemes have tried, with varying success, to provide a linguistic world-view which children can recognize. The field of reading disability has been slower to see this interdependence, but the experimental studies are now accumulating which make it clear that reading disability cannot be understood without reference to children's general linguistic abilities, especially as manifested in the period before they began to read.

Here, it seems to me, we have another exercise in looking beyond the obvious. It is fairly logical that, as reading is a visual task, we should expect to look to problems of visual processing to provide the explanation of reading difficulty (such as deficiencies in visual perception, organization, speed of processing or memory), and sometimes we do find such problems. But most 'poor readers' do very well on experimental tasks of visual processing skills, as Vellutino's review (1979) clearly shows, and other factors plainly have to be invoked. It is of course no more likely that a single explanation will be found for reading handicap than it will for any other mode of language disability. We already know that many different causes and effects need to be distinguished within such headings as 'language delay' or 'articulation disorder' (cf. Chapter 1); and when observing the angry exchanges to be found in the dyslexia literature, I have often wondered why anyone should think that this disability was any different. It is therefore encouraging to note the current research trend towards a more comprehensive coverage of the factors which have been implicated, in which an integrated account of specifically linguistic considerations seems to play an important role.

The linguistic factors are best summarized in the view that dyslexia is a 'specific' consequence of a general verbal processing deficit; that is, of a disability in one or other of the verbal coding skills necessary for spoken, as well as written language. What has to be appreciated is the range of skills involved. To be a good reader, it is argued, children need to have a good phonological coding ability, a good control of spoken syntax, and a good vocabulary range in speech, with a good awareness of the structural relationships between words. More generally, they need to have a readiness to use language (especially in unfamiliar circumstances), an ability to make their knowledge of language explicit (that is, an ability to talk *about* language), and a receptive attitude towards the language used to them, of which there has to be a great deal (as recent reports on the value of parents reading aloud to their children indicate). All of these factors are important, and they relate to other psychological skills; for example, children's ability to store and retrieve information in speech, which presupposes an adequate auditory short term memory; if this is inadequate, their ability to process language serially and hierarchically will be much affected (see also, p.100).

The consequences of this view are fairly basic. It means, for instance, that if children confuse *b* and *d*, or *was* and *saw*, we do not put this down to a simple visual confusion—if only it were so easy! Rather, it would be maintained that children do 'see' these forms as distinct (in just the way normal children do), but that they are unable to remember which verbal label is associated with which printed form; in other words, they have a deficient verbal coding facility. Years before, when they were learning to speak, they probably demonstrated a deficient coding facility also; but that kind of information is beyond the recall of most parents, if indeed they noted the difficulties as linguistic at all at the time. It is easy to notice a child's shyness, tantrums, poor coordination or difficult behaviour; much more difficult to detect that the reason for these problems may be a weakness in using or understanding ('processing', in a word) spoken language. Those studies which have been carried out do show a clear correlation between children with reading disability and an earlier speech disability. Ingram, Mason and Blackburn (1970), for example, showed that half of the children diagnosed as dyslexic had a history of deviant speech or language development, and there are several other such studies (see further, Lyle (1970), Vellutino (1979: Chapter 8), Wren (1983: Chapter 7)).

But a question arises: why not *all* the children in such studies as Ingram *et al.*? If I may be permitted to speculate, I would say that probably all the children *did* have some previous problems in spoken language, but that the methodology used by the authors precluded their discovering what these were. Without an extremely detailed developmental linguistic history, along the lines of the descriptive framework expounded in this book, all the relevant facts are just not known. A few basic measures will not suffice: the whole of the child's phonology, grammar, semantics and language use needs to be considered, in terms of production and comprehension, and this has never been done. Moreover, I would maintain that dyslexic children as encountered in primary schools very likely *still* manifest the residue of this earlier general linguistic difficulty; that is, they still have a residual problem of speaking or listening. It is a view which requires a few further remarks, by way of defence.

The usual objection which is raised to this viewpoint is best expressed in the words of one teacher: 'but there is nothing wrong with Johnny's speech. It is only his reading which is a problem.' There are two answers to this, one relating to the child's knowledge of language structure, the other to his ability to put his language to use. In relation to the first point, we need to recall a basic principle of linguistic profiling (cf. Crystal 1982a: Chapter 1): it is always easier to spot what P does say than what he does not say. It does not take a degree in clinical linguistics to observe that there is an error in the sentence *me went home*. What is much more difficult is working out which sentences, sounds or vocabulary P is *not* using, in his everyday speech. Just because T has not noticed any major error-patterns in Johnny's speech does not mean that his spoken language abilities are normal. Johnny may well be 'avoiding' the use of certain structures in speech, because he 'knows' they are difficult. It must be remembered, in this respect, that the learning of spoken grammar does not cease at age 5: many of the more advanced constructions of the spoken language, and most of a child's metalinguistic awareness, remain to be learned between the ages of 5 and 12. I would predict that dyslexic children would have special difficulty in developing their abilities in these areas; and Byrne (1981) is one recent paper which provides evidence to support this view.

My second answer to the question is to refer to the demands of language in use: Johnny may have a reasonable command of spoken language in the playground or at home, but how good is he at using his speech and listening skills when the pressure is on? How good is he at using or responding to complex verbal instructions, in tasks of increasing psycholinguistic complexity? My prediction would be that Johnny's speech is a little like an injured leg: it holds you up while you are using it normally, but as soon as you put too much weight on it, it gives. What happens when Johnny is put under linguistic pressure in this way? Does his speech not become more non-fluent than those of his peers who are good readers? There are many worthwhile hypotheses to investigate in this area, but they cannot be investigated by psychological and educational methods of enquiry alone. Dyslexia studies need a descriptive linguistic datum too.

In short, the discipline of P description, with its emphasis on good transcriptions and a hierarchical analytic approach, is an essential early step in clinical linguistic study, not simply for its potential empirical contribution, but because it can also draw attention to important issues in research theory and method. However, it is by no means the whole story, as the investigative procedure outlined on p.31 indicates. We need to move on to the more intriguing areas of analysis, assessment and diagnosis, and produce some explanatory hypotheses which will account for the data, and the sooner this can be done, the better for everyone. But we have to be cautious about embarking too soon on the theoretical road. If we approach a sample selectively, thinking that we know in advance what we are looking for, the game is lost before it is begun. And even if we begin the task of description in an open frame of mind, the pressure to opt prematurely for a theoretical decision about the pattern in the data (in effect, a linguistic diagnosis) does not go away. Anyone who has begun the task of description will know what I mean: within a few lines, a pack of hungry, competing theories grab at you, all generated by the close attention being paid to the data. It is always tempting to give way to the first insight, and follow it gratefully; but that road is the one where angels fear to tread. That way be dragons.

4

(Clinical) psycholinguistics

The descriptive aims of clinical linguistics, as currently practised, focusing on the phonology, grammar, semantics and pragmatics of individual Ps, provide us with a foundation for our study of language handicap, but they also constitute a limitation which it is important to transcend. From the study of individual Ps, it is important to move on to groups of Ps, generalizing the descriptions, and approaching a concept of linguistic diagnosis. Further, clinical linguists worth their salt would not wish to stop with their own language, but would want to compare the descriptions of P behaviour in other languages—and, in theory, in all languages—with the aim of identifying universals of language breakdown. To take just one example, is the telegrammatic speech encountered in English aphasics the same kind of thing as that encountered in French? And what is the equivalent of telegrammatic speech in languages where there are no grammatical words to leave out? It ought to be possible to say what happens when a linguistic system breaks down, or fails to develop—*any* linguistic system—and it is the aim of clinical linguistic theory to provide an explicit account of the linguistic factors involved.

But the more we see patterns across Ps, or across languages, the more we have to relate these patterns to other kinds of factor. An 'explanation', couched in the terms of a narrow conception of linguistic structure and use—phonology, grammar, etc.—will not satisfy the clinician or teacher, who has to deal with the 'whole' individual. It is always illuminating to show how there are linguistic principles operating in a mass of messy data, and, for some kinds of linguist, that would be enough. But clinical linguists cannot stop there: they must consider the medical, psychological and environmental factors which may be contributing to P's handicap, and try to see relationships between those factors and the linguistic symptoms observed. At this point, therefore, they must invoke the broader conception of linguistics, which includes a range of interdisciplinary subject areas, such as neurolinguistics and, especially, psycholinguistics.

Psycholinguistics

Hybrid academic disciplines are at once the easiest and the most difficult entities to define. It would be easy enough to refer to psycholinguistics as the study of the interaction between 'psychology' and 'linguistics', or 'psychological behaviour' and 'linguistic behaviour', and this is what some definitions do: 'the study of the relationships between language and the behavioral characteristics of those who use it' (*The Random House Dictionary*). But this does not get us very far. It leaves open the question of the 'direction' of the study. Is psycholinguistics primarily (a) the study of psychological behaviour, using linguistic theories and techniques of analysis, (b) the study of linguistic behaviour, using psychological theories and techniques of analysis, or (c) both of these? It also leaves open the question of how much of the two contributing disciplines is involved—all of psychology, and all of linguistics? Or only certain aspects of the possible relationships between these fields? In principle, one imagines that psycholinguistics, as an academic discipline, would aim to be comprehensive and systematic in its coverage of the relationships between psychology and linguistics. In practice, familiar limitations—of time, personnel and money, and the technical impracticability of researching certain kinds of topic—as well as the special influence of certain themes and personalities in the recent history of ideas have led to the emergence of a discipline which, after 30 years of development, is still fragmented and unbalanced in its coverage of the subject.

A convenient approach is to take the two constituent disciplines

Table 1   The domain of psychology

Input processes
  The way in which we select information
  from our environment; how it is
  perceived, physiologically responded to,
  and initially stored
Mediating processes
  The way in which we organize
  information; how information, once
  received, is learned, organized and
  made available for future use (i.e.
  retrieved)
Output processes
  The way in which we use information
  to construct our individual patterns of
  behaviour (biological and social), in
  relation to our motives, drives, skills
  etc.

Comparative psychology
Physiological psychology
Neuropsychology
Cognitive psychology
  Perception
  Awareness
  Intelligence
  Memory
  Motivation
  Thought
  Learning
  Personality
  Individual differences
Developmental psychology
Social psychology
Abnormal psychology
Applied psychology
  Educational
  Industrial
  Clinical

---

and specify their subfields as a means of identifying the putative domain of a psycholinguistic theory. Using various conventional sources in psychology and linguistics, I would hope that the following characteristics would receive a fair measure of agreement. First, psychology, characterized as the scientific study of the behaviour of organisms (typically, man) and of the principles governing this behaviour, as the organism interacts, socially and biologically, with its environment. Table 1 provides a more detailed specification of this field. On the left of the table is a general analysis in terms of the widely used model of information processing. On the right is an inventory of the main subfields within psychology, as usually encountered in courses and textbooks. Table 2 provides a similar characterization of the field of linguistics, conventionally defined as the scientific study of the linguistic behaviour of man (linguists typically do not ascribe 'language' to other organisms) and of the principles governing this behaviour, as man interacts, socially and biologically, with his environment. In principle, as soon as any of the theories, methods or findings from within the subfields of Table 1 are brought into relationship with the subfields of Table 2, we have a psycholinguistic study. In practice, the range of possibilities has been considerably restricted, for four main reasons.

Table 2   The domain of linguistics

Language						
Structure				Use		
Phonetics	Phonology	Grammar	Semantics	Temporal	Social	Psychological
Articulatory	Segmental	Syntax	Lexicon	Historical	Socio-	Stylistics
Acoustic	Non-	Morphology	Discourse	linguistics	linguistics	
Auditory	segmental					
				Child	Ethno-	
Graphetics	Graphology			language	linguistics	
				acquisition		
Other modes of transmission (e.g. signing)						

General linguistics, descriptive linguistics, comparative linguistics.

Applied linguistics: clinical, foreign language teaching, mother tongue teaching, translating, interpreting, lexicography, etc.

(1) *Differences inherent in the subject-matter.* There are certain subfields which are unlikely ever to be brought into correspondence in this way. Most of comparative psychology makes little or no point of contact with anything going on in linguistics. Similarly, historical linguistics would find no clear equivalent subject-matter within psychology. Much of physiological and social psychology has only the remotest of connections with linguists' concerns. Psychologists rarely find themselves worrying about the field of phonetic notation, and the mastery of the ear-training and performance skills which such notation implies. At the other extreme, of course, there are close correspondences. A

course on individual differences in psychology would find much
in common with a linguist's concerns in stylistics. Perception
relates closely to auditory phonetics. Aspects of social psychology
relate closely to sociolinguistics. And above all, developmental
psychology makes contact with language acquisition. It is not
surprising, then, to find such areas providing the focus of
psycholinguistic studies.

(2) *The bias of the investigator*. When you bring a subfield from
each discipline into correspondence, several possible directions of
study emerge. As an illustration, consider the relationship
between human memory and any aspect of language structure,
such as syntax, which would be of central concern to any
psycholinguistic theory. As a psycholinguist, one would wish to
have equal knowledge of the two subfields, and to study the
relationship between them in the balanced way implied by such
definitions as 'the study of linguistic behavior as conditioning and
conditioned by psychological factors' (Merriam-Webster, *Third
New International Dictionary*). In practice, such equal knowledge
does not usually exist in one person, and as a consequence
psycholinguistic studies generally display strong biases. If one is a
psychologist interested in memory, language is one—but only
one—of the phenomena which may be investigated as a means to
this end. The linguistic features studied will be chosen because of
their relevance to psychological hypotheses, and will often, from a
linguist's point of view, seem restricted or arbitrary. Typical
criticisms would be the overreliance on a particular model of
syntax for the description of sentence structure, or the ignoring of
other levels of enquiry, such as sentence intonation or stress.
Conversely, if one is a linguist interested in the way limitations of
memory constrain linguistic performance, a similar selectivity
and arbitrariness may take place. Typical criticisms here would be
the overreliance on a particular model of memory as an explanation for performance effects, or the ignoring of other psychological considerations, such as attention or motivation. Additional,
methodological differences in approach abound, such as the
experimental tradition in psychological study, with its
accompanying statistical sophistication, and the descriptive tradition of linguistic inquiry, with its accompanying attention to

naturalistic detail, and notational sophistication. In theory, it should make no difference if a psycholinguistics textbook called *Language and Memory* were to be written by a psychologist or a linguist. In practice, two very different books would emerge.

(3) *The history of ideas.* Osgood and Sebeok defined psycholinguistics in 1954 as the study of 'the processes of encoding and decoding as they relate states of messages to states of communicators' (p.4). In 1971, Hörmann (1979: p.18) gives a similar definition: 'the relation between messages and the individual transmitting or receiving these messages'. While the definitions are similar, the subject-matter of the two books altered radically in the intervening period, due primarily to the impact of Chomsky's linguistic thinking. Greene, writing in 1972, goes so far as to subtitle her book *Psycholinguistics: Chomsky and Psychology*. In a statement which again illustrates the 'directional' issue referred to above, she says that psycholinguistics 'remains a sub-discipline of psychology . . . its practitioners believe in the value of looking to linguistics for an analysis of language' (p.13). But in fact she looks only at Chomskyan linguistics, and her whole approach is based on the assumptions and models of generative grammar. At one point, she states that psycholinguistic research 'rests on the assumption that grammars describe the linguistic competence of the language user' (p.93), but only one of the generative interpretations of this notion is expounded. Other books written in the late sixties and early seventies display the same biases, and testify to the enormous impact Chomsky's ideas had on the thinking of academic psychologists during this period. These days, the limitations of the approach are more evident, as more recent models of generative grammar come to show up the limitations of earlier ones, and alternative conceptions of linguistic analysis become known. The fundamental insights of generative grammar remain influential, but there is no longer an uncritical reliance on the specific properties of particular grammatical models, such as dominated psycholinguistic thinking in the 1960s. In the 1980s, one of the most fruitful areas of psycholinguistic study is the role of prosody in speech production and perception, but investigators who wish to work in this area have had to look elsewhere than generative grammar for their descrip-

tive frameworks, for this subject has always been neglected in generative models of language.

(4) *The influence of applied fields.* If psycholinguistics had been left to itself, as a theoretical field, it would doubtless have developed a clear identity, as a bridge between theoretical linguistics and cognitive theory, as suggested by several definitions: 'the mental processes underlying the acquisition and the use of language' (Slobin 1971: p.5), and 'fundamentally the study of three mental processes—the study of listening, speaking, and of the acquisition of these two skills by children' (Clark and Clark 1977: p.vii). But very early on, people began to expect psycholinguistics to be useful, to help solve problems in language acquisition and use. The problems were most notable in the area of language learning—primarily, in relation to speech pathology, the teaching of reading, and second language learning. And when language professionals, such as teachers and speech therapists, come to be interested in an academic subject, especially an immature one, it is unlikely that the practitioners of that subject can remain unaffected by their concerns for long. Certainly, in the case of psycholinguistics, there has in recent years been a trend to investigate a range of problems which arise neither in linguistics nor in psychology, but in fields as diverse as medicine and literary criticism. The result has been an even greater diversification of subject-matter for the subject, and a range of overlapping interpretations of what psycholinguistics is, deriving from the different perspectives of different applied areas. For many teachers, who first encountered psycholinguistics through the work of various researchers into reading, the subject is a theory of reading. I have heard some teachers talk of '*the* psycholinguistic approach' to the teaching of reading. For many speech therapists, who first encountered the subject in relation to child development, the term is synonymous with language acquisition studies.

The diversity of subject-matter can also be found in modern textbooks on the subject. De Vito (1971) refers to speech pathology in his account of the subject—naturally enough, for it was written for a series on communicative disorders. Steinberg (1982) has a chapter on the nature and teaching of reading, and also one on second language acquisition and teaching—naturally enough, for the author works in a TESL department. But in Slobin (1971), Greene (1972) or Hörmann (1979) there are no chapters on speech pathology or second language learning—again, naturally enough, for their motivation was theoretical, not applied.

The problem with applied developments in an emerging discipline is that they lack coherence and direction. The subject is pulled in various directions. Competing theoretical models are propounded whose justification is said to be 'pragmatic'; that is, useful for one applied area, but not necessarily for others. There is often duplication of research, for example, into the teaching of reading a first language, and into the teaching of reading as part of foreign language acquisition. When in addition there are variations in research method, due to the differing backgrounds of the researchers, and changes in theoretical assumptions, reflecting developments within linguistics and psychology, it is not surprising to find a situation which is, to put it mildly, confused.

Applied psycholinguistics

An important distinction, which helps to clarify some of these issues, is that between 'theoretical' (or 'general') and 'applied' psycholinguistics. The crucial difference is the use of the word 'problems', which plays no part in the definitions of the subject quoted above. By contrast, here is the statement of editorial policy of the journal *Applied Psycholinguistics*, which first appeared in 1980. This journal 'publishes papers reporting work in which applied problems are approached from the standpoint of basic research and theory in experimental, developmental and social psycholinguistics and related areas of cognitive psychology'. The further details of the kind of problems envisaged make interesting reading, from the point of view of this chapter: 'work on both normal and disordered language and communicative development in children and normal and disordered language and communicative functioning in adults'. The following topics are said to be of particular interest:

reading, writing, learning from texts and lectures, second

language learning and bilingualism, dialect and social-class differences, the assessment of linguistic maturity and communicative competence, the application of psycholinguistics to computer language design and the design of written and oral information (e.g. instructions), nonverbal communication (e.g. sign language, gestures), delayed language development, adult and childhood aphasia, reading and writing disorders, disorders of articulation, phonology, or speech sound perception, autistic and childhood schizophrenic language and disorders associated with mental retardation, environmental deprivation, motor impairment, specific learning disabilities and sensory deficit or dementia.

Several points should be noted about such a list. First, the list is not comprehensive, but is a selection reflecting the editor's awareness of what is going on in the field. There is no significance to be attached to the mention of certain topics in language handicap and the omission of others. Secondly, the list reflects the influence of the three main fields of applied concern noted above: speech pathology, the teaching of reading, and second language learning. Thirdly, the orientation of the work in this area is in the direction of theory. The aim of the subject is to explain the nature of linguistic problems in these fields, not to solve them. No doubt, the more we understand about the nature of linguistic disability, the more our clinical intervention will be successful. But it does not follow that, lacking such understanding, our clinical work is doomed to failure. It is commonplace to achieve success, without knowing quite how we did it. And conversely, it does not follow that our understanding of a particular disability will guarantee successful intervention. That is the essential difference between psycholinguistic theory and therapeutic practice.

But there is another way to put this emphasis on linguistic handicap into perspective, and that is to look at the *potential* scope of applied psycholinguistics. It is far greater than the above list of topics would suggest. Language problems requiring psycholinguistic explanation turn up in several other areas, such as the compilation and use of dictionaries, the making and evaluation of translations, the provision and assessment of foreign language interpretation, the writing and appreciation of literature, or the production and judgement of linguistic usage. Each of these topics falls under the remit of psycholinguistics, in that they have an encoding and a decoding aspect; they are candidates for applied psycholinguistic study because they present as problems. Is the dictionary typographically clear and aesthetic? Is its information well organized? Does it meet the needs of the user? What factors led a writer to construct a poem in a certain way? What factors constrain the reader of a poem to evaluate it in a certain way? There could be a psycholinguistic theory of literature, and one of lexicography, alongside the more familiar theories of learning. One could even speculate about the relationships there might be amongst them all. It is possible that what we learn from our literary investigations might assist us in our clinical work, and vice versa. After all, the notion of 'deviance' is a topic both fields have an interest in elucidating.

The relationship between these various fields is outlined in Table 3, which should be seen as the relevant perspective for a more detailed consideration of one of the subfields: clinical psycholinguistics.

Table 3   The domain of psycholinguistics

Linguistics (study of languages and language universals)		Psychology (study of behaviour and underlying principles)			
Psycholinguistics (study of the processes governing linguistic behaviour)					
Applied psycholinguistics (study of the problems in learning and using language in the light of these processes)					
In speech pathology	In dictionary-making and use	In translating and interpreting	In literary style	In reading	etc.
'Clinical psycholinguistics'					

Clinical psycholinguistics

Ervin-Tripp and Slobin, in a 1966 review, referred to psycholinguistics as 'a field in search of a definition'. Psycholinguistics has a definition now, though it still lacks an agreed set of investigative procedures and a coherent theory. 'Clinical psycholinguistics' is in the opposite position from that of its mother-subject 20 years ago. Here, we have a definition in search of a field. For example, on the basis of the frame of reference discussed above, a reasonable definition would be: 'the study of breakdown in man's linguistic behaviour, and of the principles governing this breakdown, as he interacts, socially and biologically, with his environment, and especially, with his clinician (or teacher), clinical (or teaching) materials, and clinical (or educational) settings'. But there is no recognized training or literature which relates to the focus of this definition. Practitioners of different disciplines investigate aspects of the field—speech pathologists, linguists and psychologists, in particular—but each group has different ends in view, and uses different techniques to achieve those ends. If 'clinical psycholinguists' are not to become all things to all men, their role must be carefully identified, vis-à-vis the other professionals who have been around longer. What would a clinical psycholinguist's job description look like?

Compared with the role of clinical linguistics, clinical psycholinguistics is evidently a far more general subject, in that it takes into account from the outset the relationship between linguistic behaviour and such psychological factors as memory, attention and perception, in attempting to explain language breakdown. We are all familiar with the complex interdependence between these variables, as manifested in children and adults. Clinical linguists can describe the patterns of linguistic disability which emerge, and sometimes can explain the nature of P's handicap purely with reference to their procedures. But, more often than this, the explanation of P's handicap lies wholly or partly elsewhere—in a disordered short-term memory, or in emotional disturbance, for example. In such circumstances, the clinical linguist's account will not satisfy, and a more general perspective must be achieved. It is this perspective which clinical psycholinguistics aims to provide.

As an example of this interaction, let us consider the case of children who, after a period of severe language delay, have mastered the rudiments of simple sentence formation, and have begun to put clauses together into complex sentences, using connectives such as *and* or *'cos*. At this stage in development (Stage V on the LARSP chart of Crystal, Fletcher and Garman 1976), certain difficulties regularly emerge. The child may be able to say (or be making only minor errors in) such sentences as *The dog chased the cat* or *The cat ran in the road*, but they have problems in connecting or sequencing these within a single sentence, as in

The dog chased the cat and the cat ran in the road.
The cat ran in the road because the dog chased it.
When the dog chased the cat, it ran in the road

Typical errors made by these children can be classified into several kinds, of which the most important seem to be:

(a) The omission of elements of clause structure in the second (or later) clauses, as in

The dog chased the cat and the cat in the road.(verb omission)
The dog chased the cat and ran in the road. (subject omission)

Sometimes, elements of clause structure are omitted or obscured in the first clause, as in

The dog chased and the cat in the road. (object omission from first clause, verb omission from second)

(3 syllables) the cat and the cat ran in the road.

(b) Phrase level errors, which the child had learned to avoid in simple sentences, reappear, as in

The dog chasing the cat and cat runs by a road. (auxiliary verb omission in first clause, article omission, tense error, preposition error in second clause).

Problems in the verb phrase (with auxiliary and copula) are

particularly noticeable.

(c) The expected ratio of phrases to clauses is disturbed, in that there are fewer expansions of clause elements, especially in subject position, as in

Dog chasing the cat and cat ran in the road. (no subject expansions in either clause)

In severe cases, expansions all but disappear, reintroducing the 'telegrammatic' style of an earlier stage of language development, as in

Dog chase cat and cat run in road.

(d) Word-endings tend to be dropped, especially in the verb phrase, as illustrated by the previous sentence.

(e) Word-order may be disturbed, either slightly or severely, as in

Cat in road is running.
The dog and a cat and run in the road chasing.

(f) The whole output is accompanied by non-fluency, from slight to severe, involving erratic pauses, segment repetitions and prolongations, loudness and tempo variations, and especially abnormal intonation structuring, as in

The . the . dog chased a . c-cat . . .

The non-fluency is especially found early on in the clause, especially on subjects.

(g) Segmental articulation may be disturbed, with abnormal substitutions and omissions which are often described loosely as 'dyspraxic tendencies', as in

The [kɒg] chase a cat and a [ka] ran in [ən drɒb].

Parts of the sentence may be wholly unintelligible. Often, the subject pronoun is so weakly articulated that it is difficult to be sure which one is being used (or whether there is one there at all), as in

[ʒ] *ran in the road.*
Other unstressed grammatical items show similar weaknesses.

(h) There is a reliance on more primitive structures and lexical items. For instance, a child who had previously regularly used adjectives inside noun phrases, regularly omitted them at Stage V, or strung them together loosely at the end of a clause, as in

The dog chase a cat and angry.

The usual lexical strategy is to replace specific lexical items by deictics, as in

He chase him and it ran in the road.
He do that and it go there.

(i) Stereotyped grammar and lexis is often in evidence, especially in adult aphasic Ps at a similar stage of re-learning, as in

The you know dog is sort of chasing a cat really. . .

There may be overuse of a small range of lexical items, especially verbs which from a semantic point of view are fairly 'empty', e.g. *put, do, got.*

(j) Even when grammatical output seems to be developing quite well, there are problems of comprehension, especially in relation to clause sequences. Ps are typically unable to carry out sequences of instructions in the correct order when these are presented as complex sentences, using *after, before, when,* etc., as in

Before you give me a pen, put a pencil on the table.

These ten characteristics identify what I have begun to call 'Stage V syndrome', found primarily in older children with a history of language delay, but also encountered in other categories of P. A detailed description of the grammatical features of one such child is given in Crystal (1982a: p.46), and a fuller account will be published in due course. For present purposes, it is enough to draw attention to this putative linguistic syndrome, noting that its identification is possible through the use of purely linguistic techniques, as the examples illustrate. The *explanation* of the syndrome, however, requires a psycholinguistic investigation. Plainly, the increased complexity of Stage V sentences is somehow 'overloading' these Ps (cf. p.105). They can cope with so much grammatical, lexical and phonological complexity at a time, in single-clause sentences; but as soon as clauses have to be compatibly sequenced into larger constructions, there is a breakdown. What, then, is being overloaded? The most obvious hypothesis would seem to be P's short-term memory, though factors to do with perception and attention also need to be considered. The facilitating effect of a structured teaching environment will be a relevant factor, as will P's motivation to learn. Personality, too, is part of the picture, with outgoing children more readily attempting such sequences and encountering a different range of problems than their more withdrawn counterparts. The investigation of these factors is of course routine in speech therapy, as part of assessment and remediation, but the aim there is to intervene and obtain progress. The psycholinguists' aim is not so vocational: they wish to study these factors also, in order to understand the reasons for the linguistic handicap. Their aim is to model P's language behaviour (cf. De Vito's (1971: p.9) definition of psycholinguistics as 'a model of language performance'), and thus to *predict* this behaviour, in the light of P's other behavioural abilities. Clinical psycholinguists, *qua* psycholinguists, will stop their investigation, once they can model Ps' performance in this way. They will not attempt to do anything about it. That they leave to others, such as speech therapists and teachers, with their own range of special skills.

There is, then, a clear division in principle betwen clinical psycholinguistics and speech therapy. In practice, the division is sometimes obscured by individual personalities and clinical settings. Many clinicians nowadays have been trained in psycholinguistic theories and techniques, and use them routinely in their work. This is obviously beneficial, for the more a 'working' clinician can inform his therapy with principles deriving from psycholinguistics, the more systematic, economical and effective that therapy is likely to be. The same would apply to remedial language teaching in schools. But there is no identity between the two roles. A clinical psycholinguist is not a speech therapist or a remedial language teacher, nor is the reverse the case.

This point also emerges if we approach the study from another angle. Clinical psycholinguistics has to be kept apart from the remedial professions, because the professionals themselves form part of the object of clinical psycholinguistic study. The reasoning proceeds as follows. Let us assume that the chief aim of clinical psycholinguistics is to explain the nature of language handicap, in all its forms. This requires the systematic observation of P behaviour in a wide range of tasks and settings. By the nature of things, these tasks and settings will be predominantly clinical, introduced and monitored by clinicians and teachers. And here we encounter a major theoretical problem. The avowed intention is to model P's performance, but for the most part, spontaneous performance is absent from these Ps. Most language-handicapped children are reluctant to use whatever linguistic skills they have acquired; and most language-handicapped adults present with similar difficulties of language use and control. T's role is to elicit language from Ps who are unable or unwilling to speak, and to control the quality of language once elicited. By the judicious manipulation of remedial materials and settings, and their own linguistic stimuli, Ts aim to be sufficiently in control of P's language that systematic progress becomes possible. Without T's guiding role, so it is argued, Ps would not achieve their full linguistic potential, nor would this be achieved in a manner which would minimize the unhappiness of all concerned—P, parent, or next of kin.

The problem, then, can be summarized in the form of a question: how near can we get to an account of P's own linguistic ability, when most of the data we can obtain is the result of structured intervention on the part of T? Or, putting this another way: whose performance are we modelling, when we study clinical interaction—P's or T's? When carry-over is achieved from the clinical setting to P's natural environment, the problem disappears. But we all know that carry-over is one of the most difficult things to achieve, and one of the most difficult achievements to prove, in view of the well-recognized problems of observing Ps outside the clinic (see further, p.106). So, for the most part, we are restricted to data derived from clinical settings. The clinical psycholinguist is therefore faced with the task of disentangling those aspects of Ps' linguistic behaviour which are genuinely under their control, and those aspects which can be triggered only when the clinical situation is right. To do this, analysts need to study the way T speaks and behaves as well as P. Only by fully involving T in their observations can they explain Ps' progress or lack of it. And a similar set of arguments applies to the nature of the materials Ts use, and the settings in which they work. These arguments will be reviewed further in Chapter 5.

When we compare the aims of clinical psycholinguistics with the achievements of psycholinguistic studies in general, it is evident that there is an enormous gap which remains to be bridged. The textbooks on psycholinguistics contain a variety of subject-matter, of varying degrees of relevance. Thus the books referred to earlier in this chapter deal with the following topics: behaviourist and mentalist theories of language (usually expounded historically); the general nature of language (competence, creativity, universals, intuitions—often contrasted with animal communication, semiotic behaviour, or information theory in general); a specific linguistic model (usually the 1957 or 1965 models of generative grammar, with some reference to more recent semantic theory); a general discussion of the nature of meaning; a discussion of psychological reality (again, usually expounded historically); a developmental section, in which stages of language acquisition are reviewed and relevant theories (Piaget, LAD, etc.) recapitulated; a general discussion of language in relation to thought, culture and the world; sentence production and comprehension; speech production and perception (especially with reference to phonetic and phonological factors). A great deal of this would of course have to be covered in any textbook on clinical psycholinguistics, but there are many topics, implicit in the above discussion, which receive no mention, such as (from psychology) a discussion of task effects in relation to language (cf. Cocking and McHale 1981), or of social psychological factors as these manifest themselves in clinical settings (cf. Argyle 1967); or (from linguistics) a discussion of techniques of ascertaining linguistic acceptability (cf. Quirk and Svartvik 1966), or of socio-/ethnolinguistic studies of interaction (cf. Gumperz and Hymes 1972); or (from speech pathology) a discussion of clinical testing, as operationalized in the various procedures used with adult and child Ps. The absence of a neurological (strictly, neuropsychological) perspective is also notable in the general psycholinguistic literature, and this is something which would have to be made good in any approach devised to satisfy the requirements of a clinical psycholinguistic theory. It will make a fascinating textbook, when someone dares to write it.

5

Closer encounters:
from theory to practice

A psycholinguistic perspective brings us much closer to an understanding of language handicap, but the kind of general diagnostic observations made in Chapter 4 are still some way from the everyday tasks of specific remedial intervention. If the aims of clinical linguistics are to be achieved (cf. p.31), the gap between theory and practice has got to be bridged. How is this final encounter to come about?

Hypothesis-testing and interaction

The first step in the process is to adopt the view, now widely promulgated, which conceives of therapy or teaching as a hypothesis-testing procedure (see, for example, Aram and Nation 1982, Wren 1983, Miller, Yoder and Schiefelbusch 1983). The hypotheses about P's language handicap are generated by the theoretical models we construct, as part of our studies of normal language acquisition, short-term memory, and the like; and an attempt is made to *predict* P's behaviour, on the basis of an analysis of a sample of data, using such models. To illustrate this kind of reasoning in action, let me refer back to the Stage V syndrome outlined in Chapter 4. One of the characteristics of this syndrome is the mismatch between the phrase structures used in simple sentences and those used in complex sentences; for example, a Stage V child might be able to use an adjective-noun construction in a simple sentence, but would show no sign of this in complex sentences. Imagine now a sample of data containing sentences such as *That's a blue car*, and attempts at complex sentences in which adjectives were conspicuous by their absence. This observation would be one of the pieces of evidence leading to the hypothesis that we were dealing with a Stage V child. But how to prove it? The lack of adjectives in the complex sentences might be accidental. To check the point, it would be necessary to elicit adjectives in the complex sentence—first, perhaps, in the subordinate clause alone, and then in the subordinate clause accompanied by the main clause. A story might be constructed in which a man falls over when he sees a red car but not when he sees a blue car, and having established the alternatives, T might in due course ask P appropriate questions designed to elicit such responses as *when he sees the red car*. If P is a Stage V problem, these questions will succeed in eliciting *when he sees the car*, or the like, but the adjective will not be spontaneously used. When pressed, using forced alternative techniques (*what sort of car—the red car or the blue car?*), P will attempt the appropriate response, but will produce it in a non-fluent way, or evade the question (e.g. *that one, number two*), or display confusion in other aspects of the sentence structure (e.g. *wh—when—when he see the red car, when sees red car*). Using such criteria as quantity and type of non-fluency, or the range of grammatical errors used elsewhere in the sentence, it would therefore be possible to verify the hypothesis that the introduction of adjectives into clause structure when the sentence is complex causes specific production difficulties. And if the hypothesis was verified, it would then prove possible to talk predictively about P's behaviour. It would be possible to *make* Ps non-fluent, for example, simply by asking them to produce a complex sentence with adjectives in; and conversely it would be possible to predict a better performance by eliciting complex sentences which do not contain adjectives. In principle, it is possible to achieve this kind of confidence in relation to all aspects of language handicap, and we should certainly aim for nothing less—even though in practice, all kinds of complications ensue which make the exercise easier to explain than to implement (such as a point-blank refusal by P to do anything, adjectives or no!).

The hypothesis-testing approach to teaching can of course be illustrated from any area of linguistic enquiry (for a further example, see Crystal 1981: pp.116ff.). It is moreover widely practised, at least in an informal way, in clinical work. I do not therefore illustrate the approach for its originality, but to show how the use of predictive methods forces us to look systematically at all the variables in the clinical environment, and insists on proper account being taken of the way P interacts with T: the apparent lack of a linguistic contrast in P's language makes T react in a certain way, and the manner of this reaction acts as a check on the validity of the initial observation. In this way, clinical practice itself contributes to the process of differential diagnosis, in a manner which seems to have few parallels in other domains of human handicap.

But this way of proceeding carries with it several changes in research emphasis, whose implications need to be carefully considered. The first, and the most basic, concerns the role of T. It is no longer going to be possible to leave T out of consideration, and to study a language handicap 'isolated', as it were, from the clinic or classroom where it will ultimately be dealt with. As already pointed out in Chapter 4 (p.101), any account of language handicap cannot be satisfied with a 'pure' statement of the nature and severity of a condition, based on P's symptoms alone. It must include the analysis of T's interaction with P—in other words, of the various strategies of treatment or teaching, seen within the context of a general philosophy of management. The reason is simple: it is only by studying the results of this intervention that the validity of any diagnostic hypotheses can be properly evaluated. It is T who has to structure the environment, sometimes in order to get any data out of P at all, sometimes in order to control the flood of data which many Ps too readily produce. This structuring, with its foundations in the varying attention, memory, personality, stamina and other characteristics of P (or, for that matter, T), inevitably becomes part of our operational definition of the handicap. It thus needs a clear place in any model of linguistic handicap which we may construct.

Language handicap, in short, is an interactive phenomenon, and needs to be studied in interactive terms. This, however, is not the traditional approach to the subject, which sees a handicap as if it had some kind of independent existence—as if language delay, or an articulation disorder, resided 'in' P, and could be observed from afar, as one might watch someone with only one leg. But language handicap is quite unlike most other forms of handicap, in this respect. There is no way of knowing whether the last person you passed in the street has a language handicap or not: apart from the case of Ps who use instrumental communication aids, language handicap does not show. The only way you know that someone has a handicap is—to talk to them. Then, whether the problem is one of production, comprehension, voice, fluency, or whatever, it will become apparent. Without this interaction, you will never know.

Of course, if we had a clearer understanding of the medical, psychological, social and other factors underlying P's condition, things might be different; but we do not. In the vast majority of cases presenting with language problems, as we all know, there is no clear aetiology, and even when clear medical factors are present, there is never a one-to-one correlation between these factors and the linguistic symptomatology (cf. p.75). We are stuck with P's behaviour, and all we can hope to do is meticulously describe it and interfere with it, in the hope of controlling it, and thus explaining it. The medical factors are important, in that they provide us with a sense of P's physical limitations, and these will constrain our remedial decisions; but they do not directly contribute to remediation, in the sense of providing T with guidelines about what to teach next, and why. It is this framework of reason which needs to develop as part of the routine of clinical intervention in language problems, as opposed to the arbitrariness which all too often exists. I see no point in developing a theory of language pathology which does not take this into account.

Given this perspective, I am struck by a curious omission in the proceedings of research conferences in the field of language disability in recent years—the almost total absence of research into the characteristics of T's language. There have been several interesting papers on the characteristics of motherese, comparing normal and linguistically disabled children; but the comparable characteristics of 'therapese', and the very difficult question of how this relates (or should relate) to motherese, have been largely neglected. There are certainly important distinguishing features of clinical or teaching discourse, such as the use in early treatment of the three-part conversational turn, as in

T   What's that?
P   It's a car.
T   Very good.

or the use of overt strategies of imitation and prompt (see further, Crystal 1981: Chapter 6). Then there is the question of how P views T and the tasks provided. The point has frequently been raised in child language studies in recent years that many experimental findings can be vitiated by our failing to take into account the children's judgement as to what they think we are about. 'Why *are* these people asking such silly questions, to which (if they are normal adults) they must know the answers?' The point applies equally to the language handicapped population— and moreover to adults as well as to children. 'What then is a naturalistic environment for an aphasic patient?' asks J.M. Wepman appositely, in a discussion following a paper of Jakobson's (1971: p.326). And in relation to this, we might also ask, what presuppositions does an aphasic patient bring to the clinical setting? I am reminded of a scene in *Wings*, the radio (later stage) play by Arthur Kopit, where the heroine—an aviatrix—recovers consciousness following a stroke. She is greeted by clinicians asking her such questions as 'Who is the President of the United States?' Only enemy intelligence officers would be asking her such questions, she reasons, and so she 'decides' to say nothing. The clinicians, observing her silence, conclude that she has not understood a word they have said! Seeing a reason for a question is often part of the information needed in order to know how to answer. Failure to elicit a structure may tell us more about the limitations of our eliciting strategies than about P's structural abilities. A lack of interactive awareness may well account for some of the inadequacies found in Ps who try to respond to question batteries in conventional tests. Failure to respond is generally assumed to be lack of competence on P's part, but the interactive approach forces us to evaluate the competence of everyone involved in remediation—the test designer, materials inventor, and T, as well as P.

These are interesting theoretical and methodological questions, but at present it is the empirical weakness in the field which most concerns me—the lack of descriptions of what Ts actually do with Ps, and the lack of evaluations of how successful they, and others, think they have been. This is naturally a sensitive area, relating as it does to judgements of professional competence, but it is an area which must be properly addressed, if the remedial language professions, and the research studies which feed them, are to be taken seriously. In a frugal climate, there is no shortage of people ready to make cuts in health and education services; and if a subject is to be judged by its results (or research by its social relevance), then we must be prepared to ask these questions coolly. The required evidence, it must be remembered, is not simply that Ps have made progress (for they might have done this had they not had any remedial intervention), but that the progress was due to T, and moreover that this was due to the training which qualified T as a clinician or teacher in the first place. The remedial world is full of gifted individuals, who would be able to put plosives into a phonologically delayed parrot, if they wanted to. Their charisma would motivate anyone to learn anything. But in the search for objective evaluation of remedial strategies, these gifts are an impedance. We need to be sure that a strategy works in its own right, and not because of the personality of the purveyor. Penicillin still works, even if prescribed by a bad-tempered physician. So too we need to establish an objective causal chain of events, as part of the explanation of the nature of language handicap.

There is, then, a certain element of paradox in our enquiry. We wish to investigate language handicap, but can do this only by the simultaneous study of the clinical setting, and of T's role in particular. However, we have no guarantee that Ts will be performing effectively on any given occasion, due to their limited knowledge of the nature of the handicap they are having to deal with (and, of course, the possibility that they may be having an off day!). All too often we are having to work in the dark with language handicaps, and there is no certainty that the measures we introduce are correct, or even relevant to the condition. In which case, it is always possible that the data of disability—in effect, what we have constrained P to say, in our teaching session—may produce a quite distorted picture. If we decide to work on pronouns, let us say, we shall elicit a picture of a pronoun-deficient P; whereas if we had worked on adjectives, an adjective-deficient P would have emerged. Nor does time necessarily eliminate this bias (at least, not in the short term): progress in pronouns in week 1 will motivate further work on pronouns in week 2, and so on. It is not easy to step back from our areas of progress and begin work on other areas; but of course if a balanced developmental ability is to emerge, this must be done. (It is here that profiles of development come into their own, as they quickly indicate the gaps as well as the strengths in P's linguistic skills.) A major research initiative, then, must be made into the whole methodology of data collection and evaluation in this field, in order to be sure that the bridge between routine clinical practice and research endeavours rests on secure foundations.

The moment of truth

It might be thought, from the above account of the hypothesis-testing approach, that a bridge between theory and practice has at last been constructed. In fact, there is still a small but significant gap, and unless we can eliminate this, our bridge remains tantalizingly unbuilt—so near, and yet so far. The gap is illustrated in the discussion of the Stage V sentences on p.105 by the way I casually moved, without comment, from the abstract world of 'adjectives' to the concrete story of a man falling over when he sees a car of a certain colour. This jump is the final step in the whole clinical linguistic process. On what grounds did I move from 'adjectives' to 'colour adjectives', and moreover to two particular adjectives, *red* and *blue*? On what grounds did I feel it appropriate to introduce a man and a car, and the concept of falling over? Might the choice of these notions interfere with the adjectival hypothesis? And if the aim of the exercise were to make a recommendation to T about what to teach next, would we be able to say with confidence that *red* and *blue*, in this context, were the best adjectives to begin with? Whatever the medical, linguistic, psychological, therapeutic or other reasoning we may have grappled with so far, in arriving at an understanding of P's handicap, as soon as the decision has been made to intervene, the light from all of these domains has to be fused into a single intense beam, in order to provide an answer to the question: which actual word, or set of words, should T teach first? If the decision has been made to teach plosives, then which plosive contrast in which position in which word-pair? If the decision is to teach verbs, then which verb? This is not a trivial matter. On the contrary, it is the moment of truth for everyone concerned.

The question has to be investigated in a systematic manner, just as any other area of clinical linguistic enquiry. We cannot be satisfied with an *ad hoc* answer, of the sort 'I've always found X a good place to start.' There are probably as many 'good places' as there are Ts. Nor should we be put off by the dismissive answer, of the sort 'There's no one best place to start. Ps are all individuals, and teaching has to be matched to individual needs.' Individual differences are obviously important, but they should never be allowed to take the place of group similarities. The whole point of T training, as I understand it, is to provide a set of guidelines which are sufficiently firm to be generally applicable, yet sufficiently flexible to cater for variations in particular circumstances. It ought to be possible to devise general guidelines for the pedagogical interpretation of clinical linguistic facts, which work in exactly this way.

To illustrate this possibility, let me take one of the commonest problems to emerge in the early development of grammatical ability—the lack of verbs at the one-element stage (cf. Crystal, Fletcher and Garman 1976: p.114). There are many Ps who have a LARSP Stage I profile in which nouns, pronouns, minor sentences and other forms may be present—but no verbs. This is a gap which it is important to fill, not simply to satisfy the general remedial principle of maintaining a balanced linguistic system at any given stage, but because without verbs, the prospects of satisfactory subsequent clausal development are negligible. Let us assume, for the sake of argument, that everyone is agreed (a) that P has a genuine verb weakness, and (b) that the teaching of verbs is a priority. (It would make no difference, in fact, even if people were unsure whether the weakness was genuine: in order to check the point, the same procedures would have to be undergone.) T decides to begin teaching verbs on Monday morning. So which, of the tens of thousands of English verbs, will be chosen to start with?

This is too important a question to be left to a hypothetical T. Which would *you* choose? It might be helpful to write them down, before you read on.

Let us first consider the criteria which would help us decide. There are at least eleven that come to mind, which can be divided into formal and functional types (cf. p.49). Verbs which plausibly illustrate each type are given in parentheses (but it should be noted that the categories are not mutually exclusive). Most people think of the functional criteria first, as follows:

(a) The verbs should express a clear physical action (such as *jump, kick, drink*) and not be abstract, static, vague or mental (such as *know, do, have, feel, change*). It should be noted that these dynamic verbs can be classified into several types—most importantly, into whether the action has a clear beginning-point (*open, knock*), a clear end-point (*kick, fall down*), or has no discrete boundaries (*play, run*).

(b) The verbs should be familiar to P—a notion which usually needs to be interpreted in two ways: familiar in the domestic setting (*eat, drink, wash*), or familiar in the 'professional' setting of school, clinic, or occupation (*climb, dance, write*) (cf. Hutt 1973: p.17).

(c) The verbs should be useful to P, in terms of social or academic success (see further, Chapter 6)—*drink, go (toilet), play, like, look, stop.*

(d) The verbs should be easy to demonstrate (thus *kick, catch, walk*—but not so easily *run, climb, eat*, in normal clinical settings!); there is no point in requiring that the verbs should be easy to draw—it is in the nature of verbs to be undrawable.

(e) The verbs should be easy to learn, in the sense that they are among the earliest verbs to appear in the normal language acquisition process (*go, see, got, do, give, take*).

(f) The verbs should be frequently used in adult language—which in terms of the adults P frequently interacts with, will involve motherese (*cuddle, play, smack*) and teacherese (*say, listen, show*).

(g) The verbs should have no unfortunate connotations for P—a point more important when dealing with Ps who have problems of a behavioural, emotional or psychopathological kind (*hurt, kill, crash*).

In addition, four formal criteria can be invoked:

(h) The verb should be part of a definite lexical set, so that a clear semantic contrast can be drawn (*eat* versus *drink, walk* versus *run, walk* versus *play*)—compare *climb, look, jump*.

(i) The verb should have a regular morphology—at least as regards the use of -*ing*, which is an early development (*running, eating*). This makes the stative verbs less useful (*like, smell, want, have*). Later morphological irregularities might also be borne in mind, with T preferring regular *walk, kick* and *jump* over *run, eat* or *drink*.

(j) The verb should have a phonological structure which presents as few problems as possible—single syllable verbs rather than polysyllables, or verbs with simple CV or CVC structure (*go, run*) rather than verbs with consonant clusters. Verbs which preserve basic phonological processes might be particularly useful (such as *kick*, with its identical initial and final consonants).

(k) Lastly, there is the question of which syntactic considerations we should take into account. As we are trying to make remedial sense of a grammatical hypothesis, there is more to discuss at this point. The most important factor is that the verbs should allow an easy transition to the next stage of syntactic development. Verbs which in their everyday uses are solely transitive (*catch, give*) or solely intransitive (*go, run*) are not as useful as verbs which readily permit both transitive and intransitive uses (*eat, climb*). In response to the question 'What is the man doing?', a Stage I reply with a transitive verb (*catching*) is a problem, because this usage is weird without an object; and by definition, someone who is at Stage I cannot yet cope with verb-object constructions. On the other hand, to reply with an intransitive verb (*running*), while presenting no problems of usage, does not lead to an ability which can be easily carried over into Stage II. If P is taught only intransitive verbs, when T comes to teach Stage II, where verbs have to take objects, a whole new set of verbs will have to be introduced. The use of double-function verbs (*eating*) eliminates the dilemma, for these can be used acceptably in isolation, and also with an object (*eating a cake*).

The same considerations would apply, whichever syntactic 'path' T chose to follow in later remediation—for example, if it were decided to teach verb-adverbial constructions first at Stage II, then verbs which obligatorily take adverbials (such as *put*) would be avoided at Stage I. The valency of the verb should always be a prime consideration (see further, Fletcher forthcoming). Similarly, any idiosyncrasies of syntactic or lexical construction should be checked, before deciding on a course of action: *wash*, for example, creates *syntactic* difficulties because its reflexive use is so common (*wash yourself*); *brush* creates lexical difficulties because it collocates so commonly (for the young child) with *teeth*, and this expectation may interfere with productive use.

Doubtless there are other guidelines which could fruitfully be used, but this list will suffice to illustrate the general principle. It is now possible, using these criteria, to construct a basic remedial matrix (BRM), in which values are assigned to each verb considered to be a candidate for initial teaching. Keeping a 4-year-old language-delayed P in mind, my ratings of a small selection of verbs are given in Table 4 (H = high value, an early teaching priority; L = low value, grounds for leaving until later; ? = cannot decide). The results are quite absorbing. *Go* turned out to be much higher than I had been anticipating; *kick*, much lower.

The actual process of making the decisions was also instructive: forcing myself to decide whether a verb was, say, useful or familiar, brought the problem of teaching and learning into much clearer focus. It ought therefore to be possible, using this kind of

Table 4   Basic remedial matrix for selected verbs

Criteria Verbs	(a)	(b)	(c)	(d)	(e)	(f)	(g)	(h)	(i)	(j)	(k)
eat	L	H	H	L	H	H	H	H	L	H	H
kick	H	?	?	H	L	L	?	L	H	H	L
go	H	H	H	H	H	H	H	H	L	H	L
want	L	H	H	L	H	H	H	L	H	?	L
drive	L	?	L	L	L	L	?	L	L	L	L

technique, to accumulate a set of ratings for candidate verbs, and arrive at an overall weighting, which would motivate their early or late choice in a teaching programme. The reader might care to experiment with the items in Table 5, taken from the 5+ written language word-list of Edwards and Gibbon (1964), the 6-year verb-list of Hutt (1973), based on frequency and educational need, and the most frequent verbs in a list of 5-year-old spoken vocabulary compiled by Raban (1982), using the data from the Bristol Child Language Project (cf. Wells 1980); *be* and other auxiliary verbs are excluded; * indicates items which might well belong to some other word-class than verbs (no word-count makes this clear); + indicates items appearing in all three lists (remarkably, only 6, as it happens).

Of course, all of this is programmatic, at present. If the technique is felt to be helpful, then it needs to be investigated in a systematic manner. The first step would be to determine the extent to which Ts had shared intuitions about such criteria as usefulness and familiarity. Then it would be necessary to think about the effect of certain variables, such as the type of handicap, P's age (obviously a crucial factor, if working with adult aphasics, say), P's sex (do we rate *kick* as more useful for boys?), and so on.

Other methods of rating could be tried. Above all, we have to determine the different weightings which might be attached

Table 5   Verb lists for 5- and 6-year-olds

Edwards and Gibbon		Hutt		Raban	
bring	pick	ask	roll	bang★	look★
buy	play★ +	brush	run	buy	make +
call	put	build	say +	come	need
come	rain★	catch	sew	cut★	open
dance★	read +	clean	shout	do	play★ +
dig★	ride★	comb	sing	drink★	put
do	run★	cook	sit +	eat +	read +
draw	say +	crawl	skip	find	say +
dress★	see	dance	stand	finish	see
eat +	set★	dig	sweep	gallop	show
fall★	shine	draw	swim	get	shut
fly★	show	drink	talk	give	sit +
get	sit +	eat +	tell	go	stay
go	skip	hang	think	got	stick★
got	smoke★	iron	throw	have	stop
grow	snow★	jump	tie	hear	take
have	swing★	kick	walk	help	tell
help	take	listen	wash	hold	thank
jump★	walk★	make +	write	hurt	think
like	want	paint		keep	try★
live	wash★	pass		know	turn★
look★	watch★	play +		leave	wait
make +	work★	read +		let	want
paint★		ride		like	watch★

to these verbs, when considered from the viewpoint of comprehension, as opposed to that of production. Familiarity with such verbs as *look, listen, put* and *show* is presupposed by many teaching situations, and are plainly important for comprehension work, but hardly so crucial for work on production. A further variable would be the extent to which P was being exposed to vocabulary in written materials, which often differs greatly from that of speech—graphic simplicity motivating the frequent use of such verbs as *hop* or *see*, in some schemes.

I believe that this kind of study is well worth doing. Indeed, I do not see how we can avoid doing it, if we want to verify the claims of any clinical linguistic theory, and place our remedial decision-making on a sound and consistent foundation. I have illustrated the technique using verbs; but *any* area of linguistic structure or use could be approached in this way. Doubtless it would be necessary to introduce extra criteria, according to the phenomena being studied—in phonology, for example, factors such as functional load and phonetic salience would have to be considered. The important point is that all criteria should be made explicit and be applied systematically. The issues should not simply be taken for granted, as can so easily happen when T uses a combination of intuition and traditional clinical practice to choose a verb, an adjective, or a plosive. There are signs of a more principled approach in operation these days: acquisitional and statistical criteria are quite often invoked. But neither of these is totally reliable, in our present state of knowledge (see further, p.154), and neither of them suffices, as an explanation of the problems encountered in teaching.

The provision of materials

The final step in the process of applying any applied linguistic theory is the construction of teaching materials, based on its principles and findings. It would be easy for academic clinical linguists to shirk this step, in the belief that theirs is a world of ideas, and that it is for clinical professionals to practice what they preach. But they must not. The writing of teaching materials is an essential check on all the reasoning that has taken place hitherto; they are the ultimate testing-ground for clinical linguistic hypotheses. Moreover, they are the best way of ensuring that an approach is tried against the widest possible population. It could also be said that this exercise is the most tangible way in which academics can satisfy the demands of public accountability for what they do. And if that sounds too pompous, it can be set against the remark that the writing of materials is usually fun.

But it is also very hard work. It is, furthermore, work which, for a variety of reasons, has rarely been attempted. The remediation market-place is flooded with teaching materials, but kits, books, toys, cards, pictures or programmes based on the principles of clinical linguistics are conspicuous by their absence. (The field of assessment is much healthier; there are now many linguistically principled tests, at least in the areas of phonology and grammar.) It is instructive to see why this is so.

I am sure that the main reasons are to do with the lack of dual qualifications on the part of those who study language handicap. I do not know how many clinical linguists there are in the world, but I should be surprised if they would fill a small cinema; and very few have acquired the right kind of professional awareness to enable them to develop appropriate materials by themselves. Likewise, the number of Ts who have acquired an advanced qualification in clinical linguistics would probably fill a somewhat larger cinema; but few of them have had the time or opportunity to write materials at a professional level (as opposed to inventing *ad hoc* devices for local consumption only—cf. p.27). It is a rare person indeed who has the right blend of linguistic and clinical experience, and—perhaps more important— whose output would be respected by both sides.

This is why, in my view, the best chance for the production of clinical linguistic materials comes from collaborative ventures. I can see no way in which I, as a linguist, could ever produce a successful set of teaching materials, working by myself. Because I have never taught in a school or clinic, I lack the intuitions about how to teach a topic at those levels. In the school context, for instance, I have no first-hand knowledge or experience of what would constitute a balanced, up-to-date syllabus on a topic. I have no ability to sense the factors which interfere with the teaching of a topic, such as P's fatigue, distractibility, or his preference for a certain kind of subject-matter or type of material (worksheets, models, photographs, computational aids, etc.). I do not know how much to expect of Ps; how to motivate them; how to discipline them. I can recognize these problems when I see them (on videotape), and can analyse them, and make recommendations about them. But I cannot implement these recommendations myself (cf. Preface), and life is just too short to study all facets of the problem. A collaboration with a teacher or therapist is the only real solution.

However, when we look at the remedial market-place, we find that collaborative projects are by no means in evidence—nothing really approaching the large-scale enterprises of mainstream education, such as *Breakthrough to Literacy* (Mackay *et al.* 1970) or *Language in Use* (Doughty *et al.* 1971), and little even on a smaller scale. Having now been involved in one remedially inspired project for a few years, I think I understand why this is so: it is simply very, very difficult to find collaborators whose temperaments and timetables are compatible. The history of the *Databank* project provides an illustration.

Databank is a series of 24-page information-books, published by Edward Arnold, and written by John L. Foster and myself. Foster is a head teacher, as well as an author and editor of children's books. The series is aimed at the 11- to 13-year-old curriculum, and contains such titles as *Roads, Monasteries, Light, Deserts, Food, Volcanoes* and *Parliament*. The books are written primarily to help those children in early secondary school who have difficulties with reading, and my job is to structure the language in such a way that some of these difficulties will be circumvented. Altogether, since 1979, over 20 of these books have been published. They have been selling quite well, and reaction has been generally favourable (but see p.132). So much for the basic facts. What points of interest emerge from this experience?

The first point to appreciate is the number of people involved in the collaboration who have special roles, apart from the co-authors. This can best be explained by taking some of the more difficult books, such as the science triad, *Heat, Light* and *Sound,* and tracing the stages through which they passed from inception to completion. There were no less than seven stages involved, and what should be noted, in relation to the present chapter, are the quite specific points at which I, *qua* linguist, am involved.

(1) Somebody had to choose these topics from the range of possibilities provided by the curriculum. This is the publisher's

business. He will have made preliminary enquiries, mainly through the teachers of these children, to determine what the problem areas are, and what materials would be of most value. The role of the publisher cannot be underestimated, and I do not refer here to the obvious point that it is he who publishes the materials, and plans the time-scale and extent of the collaboration (in our case, bringing the two authors together at the outset). Of greater significance is his ability to determine the value of the project in the first place—which, in the present context, means being aware of the potential of linguistic ideas in this area, and accepting the consequences that these ideas may have for the nature of the product (see 4 below, pp.122ff.).

(2) Having chosen the topics to be dealt with, the next step is to agree on the information the books should contain. And here, in the case of the science books, there is a small problem, namely, that neither Foster nor I know our facts, in the sense that neither of us has taught science at this level, and therefore does not have the ready command of the syllabus to know what should be included. It is not the basic subject-matter which is the issue— this could be gleaned from any standard textbook or syllabus outline. For the children in question, we need to know which areas of the subject pose particular difficulty, and which, there-fore, need the most careful structuring of the language. We need to know whether there are 'tricks of the trade' which can help children to develop a grasp of the concepts. Neither of us has this inside knowledge. In short, we need the experience of a science teacher, who can orientate us towards the right kind and amount and slant of information. This collaboration is essential, if our approach is to do justice to the topic, as well as to the children.

(3) The relevant information is fed to Foster, who adds it to his other information sources, lets it simmer well for a time, and then writes a first draft of the book. It is he who makes the initial decisions about what the book should contain, in terms of subject-matter, and who outlines the number and nature of the illustra-tions. It is he, in association with the publisher, who decides such matters as whether we give lengths in miles or kilometres, and temperature in Fahrenheit, Centigrade or Celsius. And above all, in relation to the needs of our intended readers, it is he who

introduces elements from outside the syllabus, to make the material more interesting and memorable. This last point requires an example, and some further background.

It is difficult enough to remember the 'hard facts' of a subject, even when you have no problems with your reading. But if reading for you is like going to the dentist, getting access to the facts is going to be even more difficult. It is commonplace with these children for them simply to give up, in attempting to read the standard texts written for the first forms of secondary schools, or for them to read mechanically, without assimilating anything. I do not blame them. I am not a believer in readability scores, for I find their quantitative measures too simplistic (see further, Perera 1982), but if they are used on science texts designed for 11-year-olds, the scores produced are usually astronomical. It is by no means exceptional to find sentences which continue for several lines, in whose structure is included difficult terminology, formulae or even diagrams. Under these circumstances, how could a poor reader ever learn?

There are two types of solution, remedial and compensatory (see p.146), both of which have their value: we can improve P's basic reading skills, and we can modify what he has to read to enable him to achieve. *Databank* adopts the latter philosophy, and interprets it both in relation to subject-matter and to language. Thus, when Foster approaches the 'hard facts' of a topic, his concern is, first and foremost, to make them appealing and easier to remember. One way of doing this is to build in a great deal of visual information, with clear captions. Another way is to incorporate into the factual material elements of drama and fiction. A good example occurs in the book on *Railways*, where underneath a picture of Cugnot's steam machine, we read:

Between 1750 and 1800, several people tried to build
a steam locomotive. This steam car was built
by a Frenchman, Nicholas Cugnot. People watched
in fear and wonder as he drove it round Paris
at 14 k.p.h. But it overturned and blew up.
They were convinced he was a dangerous madman.
He was put in prison.

Phrases such as 'in fear and wonder' are not part of the metalanguage of science or history. Nor is a dramatic interpolation, such as the 'madman' sentence. But these points can act as hooks on which to hang the more austere facts. Once I observed a teacher trying to elicit the relevant information from his class, after getting them to read the appropriate pages in *Railways*. 'Who was one of the first people to invent a steam engine?' he asked. 'The one everybody thought was mad, said one pupil. 'Yes, the Frenchman, Nicholas somebody', said another. The answers were not brilliant, but they were far better than the usual silence, said T.

(4) At this point—and only at this point—enter this linguist. My first involvement with a particular book is when Foster's first draft comes through the post. It is my responsibility to restructure the language, as required, to bring it well within the limited abilities of the children, but not to make it so elementary that they will find it puerile. We want to compensate, but not overcompensate. The language ought to be easy, but not so far removed from the language of other textbooks that the reader would be unable to make any kind of connection. What is interesting is how, in order to solve this problem, use is made of the three main themes of the earlier part of this book—the descriptive, the acquisitional, and the psycholinguistic dimensions of linguistic enquiry.

The first task is descriptive. Every sentence that the first draft uses has to be analysed, to find its potential grammatical, semantic or graphological weaknesses. The sentence might be ambiguous, or presuppose information not already expressed; a technical term might be introduced without sufficient explanation or gloss (a particular problem in the book on *Dinosaurs*); the logical sequence of the exposition might be unclear in various ways; a pronoun might have an uncertain cross-reference; features of layout might impede comprehension of the structure. Once a problem is detected, an alternative construction must be found, and this is the main descriptive part of the exercise—to bring together a good range of other candidates which express the same meaning. For example, the first draft of *Heat* contained the sentence *Things that are burnt to give heat are called fuels*. The double passive construction seemed to be an unnecessary complication, and hearing the children read this sentence confirmed its difficulty (for instance, one child read 'bound to give heat'). A list of alternatives would include *When we burn things to give heat, we call them fuels, Fuels are what we burn to give heat, The things we burn to give heat are called fuels,* and many more.

The next step is to choose one of these alternatives, for which purpose the language acquisition literature is scoured for relevant principles. Three examples:

(a) In sequences of clauses or sentences, order of mention is preserved. Thus the first-draft sentence

Between 1500 and 1550, traffic on the roads increased, as England's trade with other countries grew.

was altered to

Between 1500 and 1550, England's trade with other countries grew. Traffic on the roads increased.

(b) Lengthy subjects are avoided, and replaced by structures where the length is after the verb. The first-draft sentence

Any objects, which people agree are valuable, can be used as money.

was altered to

Money can take the form of any objects, as long as people agree that they are valuable.

(c) Cataphoric (forward-referring) pronouns are avoided. The first-draft sentence

When they vibrate, different objects produce different sounds.

was altered to

When objects vibrate at different speeds, they produce different sounds.

(the extra adverbial being introduced, when it became apparent that most of the children had no idea what *vibrating* was).

There are many findings from language acquisition which permit a principled decision to be made. Because we know that passive constructions are still causing 7- to 8-year-olds difficulty (cf. Baldie 1976), I would avoid them, except in a few well-defined (and almost stereotyped) cases, such as the use of *is called* in definitions. Because we know that object clauses are facilitated by an explicit conjunction (cf. Limber 1973), I would usually insert the conjunction (as in *Everyone thought that it was extinct*, where the conjunction-less version too often promoted the mis-cue, 'Everyone thought it was'). Most of all, I try to make explicit the conceptual jumps which more advanced reading material makes, when explaining something. It would not be clear, for example, if the explanation of the breathing process began in the following way:

> When you breathe, air is taken in through your nose or mouth. In your lungs, oxygen passes into your blood, and this process gives your body the energy it needs . . .

The expert reader can cope with this kind of exposition, because he is able to 'see' the steps in the process which have been omitted, presumably because the author felt that they were too obvious to need stating. The poor reader finds it particularly difficult to see these omitted steps, as is evident when he is asked such questions as 'How does the air get to your lungs?' or 'How does the oxygen get around the body?' It should be noted that there is no lexical carry-over from one clause to the next:

> breathe/air/nose/mouth
> lungs/oxygen/blood
> process/body/energy.

The *Databank* treatment of this sequence spells out the steps, as follows:

> When you breathe in, air enters your body
> through your nose or your mouth. The air then passes
> down the windpipe into your lungs. In your lungs
> oxygen from the air passes into your blood.
> Your blood then carries the oxygen to all parts

of your body. The body uses this oxygen
to help make the energy you need for doing things,
and to keep you warm.

The lexical cohesion of the paragraph is apparent:

    breathe...air
       air...lungs
          lungs...blood
             blood...body
                body...energy...warm

The descriptive and acquisitional steps constitute two parts of the linguist's role in structuring the language of remedial materials; but without the third, psycholinguistic step, the progress in these areas is worth nothing. Psycholinguistics in this connection refers both to the processes governing children's motivation and ability to decode written text, to read aloud, and to talk about what they have read; and also to the principles governing the way in which writers, publishers and printers encode written language, so that it can be read with facility and pleasure. Its findings are of particular relevance, for what is the point of trying to structure language well, if the sentences so constructed cannot be read, due to inadequacies of visual presentation? Several of these inadequacies are well known to teachers and researchers—for example, the problems children have in noticing and linking both parts of a written text when one part occurs above and the other part below a picture. But there are many features of typographical presentation which have not been fully investigated, and where we can only guess at what is optimal—what typeface to use, what type size, what distance to leave between lines, whether to use upper as well as lower case, whether to use open or closed 'a', and so on. In the absence of research findings, publishers rely on intuition and tradition; but the more this can be supplemented by objective evidence, the better for everyone, writer and reader alike.

Of all the factors which could influence young readers adversely, it is likely that the features of written language which are *least* like those of spoken language will be especially significant. The fact that written language has to be constructed in lines is probably the most disturbing feature, in this respect. Evidence is slowly accumulating that the way linguistic information is organized visually in lines is of considerable importance in accounting for readers' difficulties. It can be shown that the same text, identically presented other than for the places at which lines are broken ('line-breaks'), can lead to differential performance when children read aloud (Crystal 1979, Raban 1981, Moon 1979, 1981). Certain line-breaks lead to more non-fluency (and possibly less comprehension) than others. At an impressionistic level, it is widely recognized that children will have more difficulty with a layout such as

> The dog bit the
> man on the leg.

than they will with

> The dog bit the man
> on the leg.

though the tendency to stop the sentence at 'man', in this second layout, might motivate the printing of the sentence in other ways, such as

> The dog bit
> the man on the leg.

or printing the sentence on a single line. Indeed, it is the tendency that children have to equate a line with a sentence (or, at least, a coherent unit of meaning) which is the main source of disruption.

We do not know how long it takes children to grow out of this tendency. Proficient adult readers, certainly, do not have it, but can cope comfortably with right-justified text, containing breaks at any grammatical point, and even including quantities of hyphens. However, the reading patterns of the poor readers at secondary level make it clear that line-breaks still pose a considerable problem. The extent of the problem can lead teachers—even with children of age 12—to persist in using a card to cover the lines below the one the child is reading; though how a child can thereby be motivated to scan ahead is difficult to see. But without such a crude safeguard, we do not have to look far to see the way lines interfere with reading—children jumping a line, or failing to carry meaning from one line to the next.

To minimize this interference, a strict line-break principle was used in *Databank*, based on the joint criteria of semantic integrity and grammatical hierarchy. Wherever possible, a line should be coterminous with a sentence. Where a sentence consisted of more than one clause, the line-break should coincide with the clause boundary (unless a sentence-ending miscue would ensue, in which case the conjunction would be allowed to end the line). Where the line-break came within the clause, it should be positioned between clause elements—between Subject and Verb, Verb and Object, etc. Line-breaks within noun and verb phrases were to be avoided, if possible; and under no circumstances should a line end with the initial grammatical word of a phrase (articles, prepositions). Hyphenation, likewise, was anathema.

This principle is rigorously applied to all final-draft sentences, in approximately 80 per cent of cases. The reason that it is not applied throughout has already been mentioned (p.122)—the need to give Ps some exposure to the kind of language they will encounter in texts which have not been structured in any way. However, the principle is not broken at random: I would allow an unmotivated line-break in the middle of a Foster anecdote, where the content is easy; but I would not allow one in the middle of a sentence attempting to express a thorny scientific concept, such as temperature or friction. To illustrate the principle at work, alongside the linguistic structuring outlined above, here follows a sentence printed as it might be found in a standard secondary school textbook, followed by the version which appeared in *Sound*:

Based on the time an echo takes to bounce off the sea bed from the bottom of a ship, it is then possible for the depth of the water to be worked out, or the location of submarines and wrecked ships plotted.

Echoes can be used to find out the depth of water.
A sound is sent out from the bottom of a ship.

The sound waves bounce off the sea bed. The depth
can be worked out from the time that the sound takes
to travel back to the ship. The longer the sound takes,
the deeper the water is. Echoes can also be used
to look for submarines and wrecked ships.

Principled line-breaks are not the only important typographical
feature in motivating poor readers, but they do constitute the
most novel feature of *Databank* texts. Also of considerable
psycholinguistic significance is the choice of format, the result of
a great deal of joint discussion by all parties when the series was
being planned. The books had to look adult, not child-like. They
should not appear to be 'remedial', thus reinforcing the
impression that poor readers were thick. On the contrary, they
should be presented in such a way that they could take their place
as library books, a point which the poor readers themselves never
fail to spot. The full colour cover, and the index, are two
important features in this respect. The books were to be short, so
that they would not seem to be impossible to read. They were to
be accompanied by worksheets, the language of which was to be
structured along parallel lines to the main text.

This is beginning to sound like a publisher's blurb, but I do not
mean it to. My intention is only to illustrate the kinds of issue
which have had to be decided, during the course of the project, so
as to reinforce my point about the complexity and necessity of
collaboration. Nor is the story yet over.

(5) Once the descriptive, acquisitional and psycholinguistic
decisions have been made, my revised draft is returned to Foster
for discussion. In theory, he has been responsible for the content,
and I for the language. But the next step in the process shows that
this dualism is not there in practice. In the course of my linguistic
restructuring, I frequently end up altering the meaning, in a way
which is unacceptable to Foster and his advisers. Moreover, the
kind of conceptual simplification which Foster has also introduced into the syllabus, in the interests of comprehension, also at
times proves unacceptable to the specialist. A strict specialist
vetting is required, both at local level (in the science cases, by the
teacher who originally drafted the material) and by someone

whom the publisher calls in for the purpose. As a result of this, the manuscript may go the rounds again: back to Foster, for modifications; back to me, for language checking. There have been occasions when the manuscript has made three or four round trips, before everyone is satisfied. It can take three months or more, of fairly regular activity, to complete the text of one of these 24-page books. Writing a monograph on the morphophonemics of African languages is probably easier.

Incidentally, the children themselves are no respecters of the distinction between language and content. I was invited once to a school where these books were in use. I had expected only to observe, but the teacher handed the class over to me and promptly disappeared (cf. Preface). The class had been primed with questions. I don't know quite what I was expecting, nor do I remember much of what happened, but I do recall my total confusion when one lad complained that, despite following the instructions in *Light*, he still couldn't make his Newton's disc work! Linguistic restructuring was not going to be able to save me. Fortunately, after reading the relevant section, I was able to glean enough to carry out repairs. But I have never been tempted by linguistic dualism since.

(6) At this point, with everyone agreed on the text, the story might be thought to be over; but it is not. Two other collaborators are involved, and both of them have stings in their tails. The first is really a group of people, comprising the artists, picture researchers and others in the publishing house who are responsible for putting flesh on the pictorial content of the work, and generally controlling the design. Often, in books for children, the author who writes the text and the illustrator have never worked together, and may not even have met. Very early on, we learned the importance of carefully checking all illustrative material, so that it matched the text, in terms of both content and language. It is so easy to construct a mismatch, in which the picture contains linguistic information not taken up in the text, or vice versa. An example is the first draft of the section in *Volcanoes*, headed 'Where are volcanoes found?' A map of the world was drawn, and the volcanoes placed upon it. The reader is asked to find one group of volcanoes as follows: 'Start at the southern tip of South

America. Go up the west coast of South America and North America, then through Alaska and the Aleutian Islands across to Siberia . . .' The first draft of the map, however, did not have all these places marked on it. Gaps of this kind pose immense problems for poor readers. If we tell them to go through Alaska, and Alaska is not marked on the map, then they worry, and have to ask the teacher—and feel they have failed again.

The sting in the tail comes when the artist or picture researcher comes up with an illustration which, along with the text, results in too much material to fit on a page! As it was our idea to have the illustration in the first place, of course, we have only ourselves to blame. We should have allowed more room; but it is always easier to be wise after the event. We have no alternative but to revise the text, to find the extra space—and the implications of any change or deletion have to be thought through, from all the points of view discussed in (4) above. The line-breaks are the most likely to be affected, especially when unexpected things happen. For instance, we assumed that pictures of engines (in *Railways*) would generally take up horizontal space, and were thrown when the picture of Puffing Billy turned out to take up vertical space (because of its long funnel). A caption had to be reset, and each line-break checked. Sometimes the text itself has to be changed, if an impossible line-break is encountered. There is always interaction between typographic principles and linguistic structure.

(7) Finally, the book goes off to be printed. No further problems? Not necessarily. This last collaborator can promote the growth of several grey hairs. To see this, we have to remember that the current printing convention is to produce text which has been justified on the right-hand side, as in the pages of the present book. The line-break principle, however, results in the right-hand side of the text remaining unjustified—'ragged-edge', as they say. I had assumed that a general instruction to the printer to follow our layout would suffice, and there are generally no problems when the copy is set in a galley proof. But at page-proof stage, when the text and the pictures are 'pasted up' to make an integrated and pleasing whole, there can be problems. In the early days of the project, we failed to realize the significance of this final phase, and I well recall having to sit down when, in the first group

of books in the series, I opened one at random and saw hyphens! What had happened was this. The printer had found one of the pictures to be slightly too large for the corner of the page where it was designed to go. 'No problem (he will have reasoned); it is the kind of thing which happens all the time. How you solve it is by shuffling the text to give that extra bit of space. And there's plenty of white space on this copy. Look at the right-hand margin, for a start.' So what he did was reset the caption copy, with the result that a group of lines ended with hyphens, articles and all sorts, breaking every line-break principle in this book. Whose fault? Ours, really, for not ensuring that the printer knew the import-ance we were attaching to line-breaks. He was only doing his job, sensibly, as he thought. We had omitted to note that the printer is just as much a collaborator in the project as anyone else.

Ironically, in one school I did come across a happy ending to this particular story. The teacher in charge of the remedial department had attended a lecture of mine, where I had been bemoaning these problems. She told me later that they had instituted a 'find the hyphen' competition, and rarely had her class been so well motivated!

The *Databank* project has been my closest encounter with language handicap, as the Newton's disc story will have indicated. I have valued being able to work on the project, because it has given me the opportunity to put the recommendations of various bits of theory to the test. I *believe* that an acquisitional perspective is valuable in working with language problems, and collaborative ventures of this kind provide a means of informally testing that belief. I stress 'informally'. No-one to my knowledge has taken pieces of *Databank* text along with linguistically unstructured text, and formally tested the children (apart from the Raban (1981) experiment, but this was on younger children, whose reading skills were not felt to be weak). I wish someone would do this kind of thing. But I am not disturbed that at present my only 'evidence' of the value of the enterprise is through the informal world of reviews, correspondence from teachers, and (above all) the occasional reaction from children who have used the books. One teacher sent me a set of 'reviews' written by her 12-year-old class, each of whom had been given one of the books to criticize.

The gut reaction which I value most is from the lad who wrote, after reading *Parliament*: 'I did not like about politics before, but I do now I can read it.' Another valuable reaction came from a reviewer in one of the teaching periodicals, who wrote that he could not see what role the linguist had played in the collaboration, as the books were just like any other reading books, to him. He intended the remark as a criticism; but I find it the best of all compliments. When the 'linguistics' element in a remedial project draws attention to itself, it has failed.

These are the kinds of remark which convince me that, whatever the failings of this particular project, clinical linguistic principles, as I understand them, are healthy and viable, and proceeding along the right lines. And it is *I* who have to be convinced, along with everyone else, after all.

6

The long term, the short term, and the wall

In our search for an explanation of language handicap, there is a dimension which has (if this is possible) been even more neglected than the issues of interaction and intervention presented in Chapter 5. If taken seriously, it could radically alter our understanding of the nature of this handicap, our philosophy of remediation, and our research priorities. It is the longitudinal dimension.

The fundamental relevance of this dimension can be introduced in the following way. Let us imagine that, as a result of some idiopathic disease, the government of the day has accepted the argument of Chapter 1, and given the members of the remedial language professions enough time to do all the analytical work required of them. T, anxious to carry out a detailed study of P's handicap, takes a long sample of P's linguistic behaviour, and people who know P agree that the sample is representative. It is then described and analysed from every conceivable point of view, in the spirit of Chapters 2 and 3, and the results written up and summarized. Let us assume, as a result of this process, that a clear pattern of aberrant behaviour is demonstrated, within the broader perspective of Chapter 4, so that no-one is left in any doubt about the kind and degree of language abnormality present. Let us also assume that the next step in remediation is quite clearly indicated by the kind of investigations carried on in Chapter 5. Have we, in this way, reached an understanding of P's language handicap? Would we be entitled to give our findings a label, and classify P as an example of such-and-such a syndrome? Is our search for explanation over?

No way (as a 3½-year-old language-delayed scrap said to me recently). In fact, the task of diagnosis has hardly begun. All we have done is establish a baseline in terms of which it will become possible to measure the nature of P's handicap. We have taken, as it were, a snapshot of the problem; the language is there, on tape or on the page, but frozen; the only difference between it and an anatomical specimen is that it does not have to be kept in formaldehyde. The reality of language handicap cannot be captured in this way. A language handicap is first and foremost a diachronic phenomenon—the result of a failure of language to *change over time* in the normal way. The fact of change is central to our understanding of the condition, and until we take this fact into account, by monitoring it, and building it into our model of handicap, answers to our questions about diagnosis, remediation and the efficacy of teaching will remain elusive. The implications of this orientation need to be carefully considered.

But first, a hypothetical illustration of the principle. Two 5-year-olds have both been given all possible tests, and they have come out with identical profiles—let us say, a language age of 3 years is agreed. It would then be conventional to say that they were both two years delayed, and that would be the diagnosis. But this is most misleading, as can be seen if we step back a little, and view the previous history of their conditions. Six months previously, both children had undergone another battery of tests. Child A had turned out to be at a linguistic age of 2; Child B, however, had been assessed at 2½. In other words, in the six months between assessments, Child A had caught up the equivalent of a linguistic year, whereas Child B had caught up only a half-year. Two very different kinds of handicap seem to be involved. And if someone asked us for a prognosis, our replies also would probably be very different.

'Why is this surprising?' I hear some readers (especially those with a medical background) say. 'Of course you have to take the normal time-scale of a disease into account in defining its nature. If one disease takes a week to run its course, from initial symptoms to recovery, and another disease takes three weeks—all things being equal—then they would usually be considered as two distinct diseases.' Exactly. It is routine in the medical model for temporal factors to be referenced—the time between infection and first symptoms, the time sequence of symptoms, the time it takes for a drug to work, the time the body takes to recover . . .— because the theoretical significance of time is appreciated. My argument is the same: that differential rates and courses of development are a defining feature of language handicap, and that progress in the field is dependent on recognition of this point. And if I am right, this makes the almost total absence of any reference to time in the language pathology literature all the more remarkable (but cf. the excellent discussion in Aram and Nation 1982: pp.62ff.).

The diagnostic significance of time is, indeed, often *implied* in the discussion of problems. For example, estimates may be given of the time it takes for a 'normal non-fluency' in a 3-year-old to clear up: if it persists, then it is not normal, by definition. Or comments are made about certain articulatory disorders, such as that discussed in Chapter 1, being 'resistant to therapy' (p.13). Or T feels that the rate at which P is acquiring new grammatical constructions is 'rapid'. But such sporadic remarks are no sub-stitute for a theoretical perspective in which the temporal course of a language handicap is plotted, in relation to the quantity and quality of intervention provided.

The reason this perspective is lacking is almost certainly a further reflex of the problem of time in the other sense (Chap-ter 1). It takes time to study time. To produce a language learning curve for P, samples and analyses have to be repeated at intervals. Explicit, meticulous records have to be kept. It is time-consuming because a wide range of features have to be noted. It is not possible to keep a note of just a few, for the obvious reason that we do not know in advance which linguistic features are going to be the salient ones, when it comes to defining the learning curve. Which features are going to clear up of their own accord, without therapy? Which will respond best to teaching? Which will respond poorly or not at all? If only we knew in advance . . . But at present, apart from a few ill-formed intuitions that some aspects of language are more difficult to teach than others, we do not.

Research into the temporal characteristics of language handicap is of considerable practical, as well as diagnostic value. If there are, indeed, factors governing the acquirability of a particular group of sounds, grammatical constructions or lexical items, then T needs to know, in order to evaluate what it is possible to get done, given the limitations on time and resources. We need to work towards a goal where it is possible to quantify the amount of change that T can hope to introduce into P's system, given N hours a week, when working on sound X, construction Y or lexeme Z. I do not wish to trivialize the point, but there are analogies which can be drawn with largely mechanical procedures, such as building a wall. If you want to make a wall a certain height in a certain time, it is possible to work out how many bricks and how many bricklayers will do the job—allowing a little for different bricklaying abilities, and the kinds of problem which interfere with the smooth running of the schedule (such as the non-arrival of a supply of bricks). Now, without wishing to push the analogy into an early grave, there are some points of resemblance between bricklaying and language teaching. (In fact, people do sometimes talk loosely about the 'building-blocks' of language, when thinking of language acquisition.) The strong point in the analogy is the implication that there is a determinate number of teaching goals (sounds, sound combinations, lexical items, etc.), some of which have to be present as a foundation for others. The weak point in the analogy is that the bricks are not all of the same size or significance, nor is it necessary for one tier of bricks to be complete before the next tier is begun. There are also rather a large number of interfering factors, equivalent to the bricks not arriving on time. But whatever the weaknesses, I hope the analogy still has some point: T needs to think of himself to some extent as being in the position of a building contractor, who can say with confidence that, given the men available, the wall will be built in a definite number of days. Until this can be done, all the discussion of 'syllabuses' for language disorders, or of therapy or teaching 'establishment', is so much sound and smoke. How can one possibly work out how many topics to get through in a term, or how many sessions to devote to a case, or how many people to appoint in a district, if one does not know how long it will take to do the job which needs to be done? Without a clear, quantitative case, how can one convince people who are conditioned to thinking in quantitative terms? This is the weak point in all arguments about T staffing and resources, of course; for we all know that this kind of argument cannot yet be made. But unless and until we appreciate the nature of the argument that is required, how else is the required research to be motivated?

When I first propounded this argument in a public lecture, I used the title 'How long does it take to teach b?' I was not expecting the reaction I received, which was one of total incredulity that such a question could even be asked. 'There can be no answer to the question,' it was said. 'Everything depends on the willingness of the child to learn, the kind of T he has, the nature of the setting, whether parents help, the nature of the handicap . . .' But, apart from the last noun phrase in this list (which contains the fallacy, already noted, that the time factor in a disorder is somehow different from the disorder itself), these points add up to no more than a complaint that the task is a difficult one. Moreover, it is a fact that, every day, Ts act as if they *do* know the answer to the question. An experienced teacher knows that, on average, it will take X weeks to get a child from Book 1 to Book 3 of a reading scheme, and will quickly develop a sense of trouble if children take longer over Book 1 than they should. And therapists have no trouble altering their expectations of progress as they move from working with children of above-average intelligence in a language unit, to working with an educationally subnormal population in a special school. They *know* it will take longer to teach something. It is my belief that this kind of intuition can be sharpened to deal with the whole range of language handicap, and that a main aim of research is to provide the facts and criteria which will enable T to sharpen it.

The field of language acquisition research is already beginning to be helpful, in this respect. Anyone who encounters this research begins to develop a sense of norms for the learning of linguistic features, and it is possible to systematize this knowledge in the form of a developmental scale (as in our work on profiles, cf. p.20). It is already possible to say something useful, therefore, about how long it should take for a child to move from point A to point B. In recent years, it has been fashionable to stress the marvellous speed with which a child learns properties of his language. These days, there is a more sober awareness of the length of time it takes for a child to acquire perfect productive control of a linguistic domain. To take just a few examples: fricative consonants can be heard in the second year, but children of 6 or 7 still have trouble with some of them (e.g. Edwards 1974); passive constructions may be heard as early as 4 or thereabouts, but they are still being sorted out at 7 or 8 (e.g. Baldie 1976); definite and indefinite articles may be heard from around 2, but 7- and 8-year-olds still make errors of reference in their use (e.g. Maratsos 1976). It is easy to be impressed by the first signs of progress, as children start out on a language learning road; what is also important is to see the length of the road they have to travel, as they move towards the norms of the adult language.

A similar, long-term implication emerges if we look at the topic of motherese. Here, we are concerned with describing the kind of input language which children receive as they move from point A to point B, and determining what influence this language has on their subsequent performance. This reference to motherese is important, for the focus on interaction which it implies provides the most significant point of contact with T's own role (cf. the argument at the beginning of Chapter 5). If T knows how long it would take a 'normal' mother to get her 'normal' child from A to B, using a 'normal' range and quantity of motherese structures, then this knowledge can provide a perspective—it could be the essential perspective, in fact—for T's own work. At present, the motherese literature provides us more with theories and methods than with facts (see the state of the art review by Gleitman *et al.* 1984), but there are already some stimulating and not entirely expected implications available for those who are beginning to think about this perspective. In particular, this literature forces us to look carefully at the question: how long does it take for a parent's use of a linguistic feature to be assimilated and used productively by a child? There will presumably be many answers, depending on the kind of feature we are thinking of and the age of the child; but there are some interesting suggestions that the length of time may be much greater than might be expected. I asked a group of mothers how long they thought it took for their language to be picked up and used by their children. The answers ranged from minutes to days; no-one thought it might be weeks or months. Yet consider the implications of such studies as Furrow, Nelson and Benedict (1979). They investigated the speech of seven children and their mothers, when the children were $1\frac{1}{2}$ and $2\frac{1}{4}$. Several syntactic characteristics of the speech were analysed, relating to the type of sentence (statement, question, etc.) and the kinds of structure used (noun and verb constructions, word-endings, etc.). It did not prove possible to show much of a relationship between the mothers' speech at age $1\frac{1}{2}$ and the child's speech at that age, but there was a strong, positive relationship between the mothers' speech at $1\frac{1}{2}$ and their children's speech at $2\frac{1}{4}$. In terms of the measures used, the authors claimed that the mothers' speech was significantly predicting *later* child speech. Now correlations do not inevitably mean causation, and it is hardly possible to generalize, with such a small sample and such a restricted age range, but there is still a distinct implication that it may take several months for a child of $1\frac{1}{2}$ to assimilate aspects of his mother's grammar, and put it to use. And if it takes a normal child several months before the effects of grammatical input manifest themselves, we might continue to speculate, how long will it take a linguistically handicapped child?

It is at this point that we must carefully consider another of the paradoxes which pervade remedial language studies, but this one is the most curious of all: the paradox of rapid returns. It is most clearly illustrated from one of the most frequently occurring types of handicap—language delay (other categories of handicap will be referred to below). Let us take a 4-year-old with a considerable delay, such that he is using grammar, somewhat abnormally and erratically (as is always the case, for language-delayed Ps are never replicas of their juniors), at the level of an 18-month-old—Stage II in terms of LARSP, shall we say. T is approached to begin therapy. (It should be recalled, at this point, that the hypothetical government of p.133 has so arranged matters that every P has been assigned his own T, in a one-to-one situation, so problems of a practical kind should not arise.) But, wait! Let us first ask what expectations T has about the course of the therapy, in much the way P's parents might ask, 'How long will it take to make him like other boys of his age?' Ignorance would make any of us hedge, when forced to reply, and a qualification in tactful hedging is presumably a part of any good course of T training. But this is an intellectual enquiry, not a parent counselling session, so let us not hedge. Is it possible to make any predictive statements at all about P's progress towards 'normality'? The answer is yes; and the paradox is that this answer is different from what many Ts expect.

It is an axiom of remedial language teaching that structured intervention will create progress. And if the long-term goal is to get P 'within normal limits', it is moreover axiomatic that this progress must manifest itself *more rapidly* than it would in the case of a normal child at the same language age. To see that this must be so, we have only to look at the two alternatives, neither of which provide acceptable remedial philosophies: slower progress or equivalent progress. Slower progress is obviously unacceptable, as an aim—though plainly we often have to accept this in practice—for the gap between target and achievement will slowly widen. In one chronological year, P does not learn one language year. By age 5, in the above case, P might have progressed to a language age of 3: he would then be 3 years delayed, not 2. What is slightly less obvious is that equivalent progress is no more acceptable—that is, P progresses at the *same* rate as that of a normal child at the same language age, with a chronological year equalling a language year. This seems logical enough, but it is unacceptable. A moment's thought makes it clear that, on this basis, P would remain behind his peers for the whole of his language acquisition period: unless he reached a linguistic 'ceiling', he would always be $2\frac{1}{2}$ years behind. In due course, this would not matter, in theory: at 25, he would have the linguistic abilities of a $22\frac{1}{2}$-year-old, one imagines, and this would hardly hold him back. (In practice, of course, ceiling effects are extremely common, and the gap generally widens dramatically at some point.) But equivalent progress would create havoc with his school placements, in the meantime, and would place P's educational advancement severely at risk. There has to be a better way.

That leaves the first alternative: if Ts have the long-term aim of 'normality', they have to aim for P's progress to be faster than normal; otherwise, P will never catch up. There has to be a policy of rapid returns, if Ts' professionalism is to be warranted—and therein lies the paradox. Ts have to be able to say that P will move faster than normal, while being perfectly aware that the reason P is in his present position is because so far he has only been able to move slower than normal. And even if Ts do *not* believe in the long-term goal of normality, they cannot escape the pressures imposed by the paradox, for they still have to face up to the questioning of parents, who so often identify their hopes for normality with their confidence in Ts' professionalism.

How can Ts possibly extricate themselves from this mess? The most radical solution is to give up the focus on normality—a possibility we shall consider shortly. In practice, most people are reluctant to take this step, and seem to fall back on one of two solutions, if asked to provide a rationale for their work. First, they may adopt what we might call the 'all the eggs in one basket' solution. P does indeed make rapid progress, but only through the sleight of hand of T teaching him a restricted area of the language. By working intensively on X, Y and Z, rapid progress is made in X, Y and Z, and a year later, tests of X, Y and Z show that P has caught up by so many months. But no work at all has been done on structures A to W, and little of the hoped-for spontaneous generalization has taken place. This kind of practice is widespread—forced on T, often, because of lack of time, and the persistent demand for 'results'—but no-one should be fooled into thinking that it is a solution. At worst, it leads to the danger of teaching only the structures that appear in the tests. At best, it leads to a situation where P's abilities are highly selective, and where he has a limited ability to 'carry over' his skills from clinic into everyday use. Either way, it is a trap from which there is no escape. There is no solution to be found here—only more dragons.

A widely practised alternative is to opt for what we might call the 'proof of the pudding' solution. Here, any progress at all is felt to be better than none, even if it is slower than normal. The justification for Ts' professional intervention is that they have been able to promote change in P, which would otherwise not have been likely to take place (or, at least, where it would have been ethically improper to assume that it *would* otherwise take place). Everyone is doing their best. This of course is the rationale for professional intervention in the most severe kinds of language problem, such as are found in mental handicap, where the tiniest of developments can be a source of delight to all involved. But this is a short-term rationale only, which needs to be placed in a longer-term perspective if we are to provide convincing answers to the questions of curriculum and planning. It can also be a dangerous rationale to adopt, especially in cases where P has no evident major cognitive or physical deficit, for it can so easily become a convenient way of avoiding the real issues. T works hard and makes progress on a specific linguistic point, and everyone is pleased; but it is easy then to forget to think through the implications of this kind of success, in the longer term. What have we actually *done*? Will P continue to use this language spontaneously, or will T need to provide him with regular further reinforcement? Will his ability to use this new language be at the expense of an inability to do something else? Is the language we have taught a valuable foundation for subsequent linguistic work (cf. the wall analogy)? Above all, have we chosen to teach forms of the language which might act as a catalyst for his learning of other forms, without T intervention? The proof of the pudding is not in the eating, in linguistic matters. It lies in P's ability to generate further puddings.

There is a further possibility, and that is to recognize what may indeed be the only reality—that this 4-year-old P will never be normal, no matter what we do. Let us explore this possibility. 'Not normal' here must be interpreted in relation to both language structure and language use. It means that there will be linguistic features—sounds, grammatical constructions, vocabulary—which P will always inadequately command. Certain features will be used inadequately, or not at all, or be perceived or comprehended with difficulty. Depending on the speech situation, and such variables as audience, task, emotional involvement and fatigue, so the problems will be greater or less. Now, we really know very little about what happens, when language delayed children grow up. There have been very few studies. But the studies which do exist are quite unequivocal in their conclusions (though the question still needs to be investigated of how far these Ps operate 'within normal limits', compared to those of their linguistically less able peers who were not referred for speech therapy as children).

Weiner (1974) documents a longitudinal study of a boy with severe language problems over a 12-year period, from age 4 to 16. He made considerable progress, but at 16 he still presented with many syntactic difficulties. Hall and Tomblin (1978) looked at 36 adults who were language or articulation impaired as children. Those with language impairments continued to present problems. Other follow-up studies tell the same story (Wolpaw, Nation and Aram 1977, Aram and Nation 1980, De Ajuriaguerra et al. 1976, Griffiths 1969, Garvey and Gordon 1973). In their discussion of dysphasic children, De Ajuriaguerra et al. (ibid.: p.368) conclude:

> The ultimate goal of training is to bring these children nearer the norm in language as well as in intellectual mobility and affective exchanges. But is this possible? We believe that with the methods we employ, within certain limits, we arrive at substitutes rather than a reconstruction. In this frame we might ask if, instead of attempting an ideal that the child cannot attain, we might not better use tasks that are possible for him without binding him by normative values attached to standardized tests.

In Aram and Nation (1982), there is an instructive account of a 25-year-old adult whose communication handicap was first suspected as early as age 1. Despite a high non-verbal IQ, and multiple encounters with all kinds of specialists, he continued to present significant language difficulties. This is how the authors summarize the young man's position:

> Twenty-four years after his mother raised questions, Gary continues to present a host of language, learning, social, and vocational problems. Although he is gainfully employed, talks in sentences, has completed high school, and

occasionally dates, he has not grown out of or been remedi-
ated out of the language and learning problems he presented
as a young child. Although he has made immeasurable
progress, using all aspects of development as a floating
referent, he has never been able to close the gap between
himself and his peers. Gary continues to be a language
disordered child grown up. (1982: p.68)

A language disordered child grown up. I am slowly following
up some of the children who were referred to me for a linguistic
assessment in the 1970s, and though most of them are hardly into
their teens at present, the picture which is emerging is undoubtedly a similar one. While I have nothing systematic to report as
yet, I do have a relevant anecdote, which also illustrates one of
those coincidences that prove the existence of a clinical linguistic
guardian angel (as opposed to a terminological demon). While
writing this chapter, I came across someone whom we had worked
with years before—as a matter of fact, the boy who provided the
($3\frac{1}{2}$-year-old) child case study for Crystal, Fletcher and Garman
(1976). I met him and his father in the street. I recognized the
father, but not the boy. He was now 13, and quite a bruiser. He
was a bit shy—but my own children at that age could have passed
for elective mutes sometimes! We passed the time of day, and I
didn't notice anything abnormal in what he said. Indeed, I was so
busy listening to how he was speaking, my own speech probably
seemed far more warped! His father was with him, and he took me
on one side. He began to tell me how well his son was doing, and
then mentioned that he still had 'a few problems'—got a bit
tangled up sometimes, and sometimes you had to repeat things to
him. 'Mind you,' the father laughed, 'Don't we all get into a
muddle sometimes?' Indeed we do, but there are muddles and
muddles; and I do wonder how far success, in such cases, is due to
P learning to live with his handicap, rather than it being 'cured'.
If we had subjected him to a barrage of tests, along with his 13-
year-old peers, as some of the American studies have done, I
wonder how he would have fared. Not well, I suspect.

We desperately need to tighten up our understanding of this
end of the developmental scale, in dealing with language handi-

cap, so that we can become clearer in our minds about what it is realistic to seek to achieve. As Aram and Nation put it, 'One of the shortcomings in the profession of speech-language pathology has been a failure to collect and report longitudinal data', and they conclude: 'A longitudinal perspective of child language disorders is needed if we are to guide our language disordered children and their parents beyond the pre-school years' (1982: p.62). I fully agree, but I would want to extend the argument much further, to include all categories of language handicap, adult as well as child, and other categories apart from 'language disorder'. For me, the longitudinal dimension is not merely a 'perspective' for language handicap; it is part of the definition of the handicap. Moreover, it is a perspective which, if adopted, can radically alter the way in which everyone involved in language handicap carries out their work—charitable organizations, teachers and therapists, and researchers.

The charities will naturally concentrate on the broader human perspective—on helping the language handicapped to cope with the problems of social isolation (a particular difficulty for the teenage group), to help develop public awareness of their special needs in the field of further education, and, especially these days, to try to lift them out of the bottom of the pit of the unemployed. To take just this last example, if language is going to continue to be a problem, then the difficulties will manifest themselves most noticeably in situations of tension, such as job interviews. Communication is at the centre of most jobs now—even if it means no more than understanding health and safety regulations (see Crystal 1971: Chapter 1). But who is there to help the language handicapped child, once he has ceased to be a charming 'little boy' or 'little girl', and become a less attractive post-adolescent? He has been 'discharged'. He has 'left school'. His parents may no longer be so involved. And how many of the general welfare agencies know anything about a history of language handicap? Fortunately, in terms of welfare, the situation is slowly changing, at least as regards those handicaps for which there is a fair degree of public recognition, such as mental handicap and deafness. But handicaps such as language disorder and dyslexia are still some way behind. The charitable bodies, accordingly, have a major problem on their hands, in drawing government attention to the nature of the need. Apart from the inherent difficulties involved in attracting the attention of a government about anything, these bodies have difficult decisions to make over priorities. Most of the effort to date has been, quite rightly, in relation to the gaps in provision for the young language handicapped child. One of the slogans of the UK's AFASIC (The Association for All Speech-Impaired Children) is: 'a language unit in time can save expensive special education at nine'. But if your time, effort and money are focused on the early end of the developmental road, it is by no means easy to focus just as much attention on where the road is leading. There is only so much time and effort, and even less money.

The change of direction implied by adopting a longitudinal perspective for language handicap is just as significant for teaching and therapy; indeed, the implications are far-reaching. There is no need for language specialists to think this through from scratch: the basic intellectual and pedagogical implications have already been well rehearsed in relation to learning disability in general, and there are several standard discussions in the field of education (e.g. Chazan 1973). With some areas of special education, it is normal practice to accept the view that the handicapped children will not catch up, and a philosophy of compensatory education has been developed and put into practice. Those involved in language work, therefore, need to familiarize themselves thoroughly with the educational debate, as a preliminary to deciding what can and should be done in relation to their own field. Gearhart (1981), for example, draws the distinction between remedial and compensatory teaching in the following way:

Remediation (remedial teaching) includes those activities, practices, and techniques that are directed toward a strengthening of specific areas of functioning that are viewed as weak or deficient . . . [By contrast,] accommodation and compensatory teaching refer to a process whereby the learning environment of the student, either some of the elements or the total environment, is modified to promote learning. The focus is on changing the learning environment or the

academic requirements so that the student may learn in spite
of a fundamental weakness of deficiency. (p.261; see also
Marsh, Gearhart and Gearhart 1978: p.85)

These particular definitions come from a chapter discussing
teaching programmes for the child in secondary school, hence the
reference to 'student'; but the point of the distinction can be
generalized to any level of education, and can go beyond education, in the sense of academic success, to the domain of social
success generally. In the language world, the issue has already
been much discussed in relation to the linguistic needs of
immigrant minorities.

But there has been little discussion of the matter in relation to
the needs of the language handicapped child—or adult. Nor is it
known what professional opinion is on this matter. I have
therefore been making a thorough nuisance of myself recently, by
asking every speech therapist I meet whether they have a belief
that remedial linguistic intervention is likely to be successful—
that is, instil normal competence—or whether they feel the need
to develop some alternative, perhaps in the direction of compensatory approaches. I have been surprised by the consensus
which has emerged in the responses. The majority of therapists
said that they were unfamiliar with having the distinction presented to them in this way—though on reflection, this is perhaps not
so surprising, for there is a marked lack of educational (as opposed
to therapeutic) theory in training courses (I have not yet found a
remedial language teacher who was not familiar with the general
issue). But of course all were familiar with the distinction between
language structures and language use (cf. p.49), and all had had to
cope with the issue in practical terms, partly because of the need
to provide some kind of answer to the question asked by parents
or relatives, 'Will he get better?' What, then, was the consensus
which emerged?

Without exception, there was a belief in the long-term efficacy
of remedial intervention. Therapists who worked in community
clinics, or in language units attached to normal schools, expressed
the view that their job was to instil a basic 'core' of language
structure, so that in due course Ps' language skills would become

commensurate with their other (social, psychological) skills, might even aid his acquisition of these skills, and certainly would aid his educational development, by providing a linguistic foundation upon which teachers could rely, as they worked their way through the curriculum. Therapists who worked in special language schools were more cautious in their hopes, and several showed the influence of compensatory approaches, but the general view was still one of remedial efficacy, a commonly cited criterion of success being whether the child could be taught enough language to be able to leave the special school, and cope with the linguistic demands of mainstream education. Several examples were given of children who had progressed sufficiently to get to a normal secondary school, but no-one seemed to know what had happened to them thereafter. Therapists who worked in schools for the physically and mentally handicapped also expressed their support for the principle of remedial efficacy, although accepting that the severity of the condition was such that it was difficult to achieve. A general argument here was that, as we do not know the maximum linguistic learning potential of the children, we cannot dispense with a remedial aim, even though the ultimate achievement will be a long way from normal. And therapists who worked with adults, in hospitals or follow-up settings, also believed in the principle, despite the currents of criticism which have been directed towards the concept of aphasia therapy from time to time. Their reason was similar to that used by their colleagues in mental handicap: they cited the undiscovered potential of the brain, and argued that with more time, resources and knowledge, a remedial philosophy with aphasics could be successful.

Now let me be clear about this: I asked only about 20 therapists altogether, so you can take these results or leave them. What you cannot do is fail to address the question, and think out your own position, in relation to the longitudinal aims of teaching—not just in relation to the immediate concerns of clinical practice, as the therapeutic handbooks instruct (distinguishing between short-term and long-term goals), but as a philosophy. For clarity, let me restrict the discussion once again to the commonest yet least understood kind of handicap. Do you believe that the next seriously language-delayed child you see is, one day, going to 'be normal', or do you not? To avoid red herrings, let me put the question in a stronger form. Do you believe that, if you had all the time in the world, and all the resources that you needed, the child would be normal one day? I find that, when the question is put in this way, many Ts say yes. I have had to think this through, like everyone else, and I reluctantly find that, but for just one caveat, for the reasons I gave earlier, my answer has to be no.

It is an important caveat, for without it there would have been no point in writing this book, or engaging in clinical linguistic research in the first place. I have to recognize the possibility that the main reason for the long-term inefficacy of intervention, in the cases described above, may be the inadequacy of the traditional methods of intervention themselves—lack of knowledge about the best way to grade and present linguistic features, and general uncertainty about the optimal time for the teaching of particular features to take place. What we do not know, at present, is far more than what we know. And naturally, if Ps are inadvertently given the wrong linguistic medicine, their chances of recovery will be much diminished. If this is so, then we also have to allow for the possibility of breakthrough, both on the medical side and on the behavioural side. On the medical side, we cannot rule out the discovery of specific patterns of neurochemical deficiency, which would account for specific patterns of linguistic handicap, and which could be treated by pharmacological methods. Why shouldn't there be drugs which would promote the growth of language, or even particular properties of language, at particular periods of development or stages of learning? Similarly, on the behavioural side, and in the absence of medical progress, is it not conceivable that our remedial knowledge will increase to the extent that T will be able to dispense precise linguistic prescriptions, to achieve normal language behaviour?

All of this may be possible. More to the point, to keep our long-term research motivation in a reasonable state of health, we have to believe that something along these lines will happen—that in due course intervention based on sound clinical linguistic principles will reduce the problems attendant on teaching specific features of language, and promote the development of accelerated learning. It is a great act of faith, but there is some evidence already available—small-scale and anecdotal, but evidence nonetheless—to justify it. The evidence that first convinced me came from cases where traditional teaching techniques had been used for some time to no avail, and where a switch to linguistically orientated techniques proved immediately successful, within certain limits, as in the account of the aphasic patient in Crystal, Fletcher and Garman (1976). But there is a dearth of documented cases of this kind, where such techniques are shown, in the absence of any clear alternative, to provide a principled basis for intervention, or where they are shown to be efficacious, after other methods have failed; and there are no cases at all which look at the long-term consequences of the application of these ideas. This is not surprising, given the youth of the subject; but until such evidence becomes available, it is only wise to make the minimal claims for it. I therefore hope and expect that clinical linguistics will provide a breakthrough in this field, and I continue to work towards this end; but I do not assume that this *will* happen, and I certainly do not think our expectations in this area ought to blind us to present-day clinical realities. I therefore note my caveat, but do not allow it sufficient status to alter my pessimistic answer. Even with linguistically inspired intervention programmes, we may have to accept that the long-term prospects for the remediation of serious cases of language handicap are far less than we would like, in relation to the target of normality.

A lot will of course depend on what counts as 'serious', in such questions, and what will ultimately count as 'normal'—or 'within normal limits', which is a euphemism widely used in this context, to avoid having to say 'no'. These are important considerations, but they do not affect my main point, which is the need to understand the absolute limits under which remedial language teaching has to work, and the consequences for syllabus design which follow. The issue is *not* one of the number of people and resources; it is not simply a matter of time (cf. Chapter 1). It is a matter of knowing what is best to do, and what cannot be done, even if we had all the time in the world. If we cannot make the whole of P's language normal, by age 16 (or 20, or 30 . . .), then we must select those areas which we know will maximize his chances of academic, social and personal success. But what principled basis can we give to this selectivity?

This question needs to be answered in structural as well as in functional or pragmatic terms, but only the latter seem to have been addressed, as part of a weak notion of compensatory teaching. For example, it is common in aphasia therapy to devise some kind of functional framework within which the needs of P can be identified, and individual therapy initiated (cf. Sarno 1969, Skinner *et al.* 1983, Code and Muller 1983). The categories of the framework are defined in terms of language in use—the language P needs in order to achieve, such as attracting attention, requesting objects or responding to a question. With children, a similar emphasis is to be found in current work on reading ('functional literacy' programmes), on language in education (the various 'language in use' projects, such as Doughty *et al.* 1971), and on pragmatic studies of acquisition and handicap (Gallagher and Prutting 1983, McTear 1985). Now, while it is by no means easy to define functional linguistic categories in a clear and consistent way (cf. the critique in Crystal 1976: Chapter 3), or to construct a coherent pragmatic theory, it is not too difficult to produce a simple inventory of language functions which can provide a basic tool of assessment or remediation. Common sense tells us that there are a few essential communicative functions which it would be desirable for all human beings to be able to control (greeting, thanking, questioning, and so on), and it is possible to add, somewhat arbitrarily, to this list, as ability increases, in much the same way that communicative notions are incorporated into modern syllables of foreign language teaching (cf. Johnson and Porter 1983). These everyday concepts can thus provide the rationale for selecting areas on which to base a programme of pragmatic teaching, whether we are dealing with adult aphasics or pre-school, language-handicapped children. For children in school, the rationale is the same, except that it will be more influenced by the functional categories constituting the curriculum (mathematics, English, science, religion, etc.).

But what comparable rationale is there for selecting the aspects of language structure to concentrate on, in an intervention programme? In the field of grammar, for example, which structures can be said to be more important than others, from the point of view of both short- and long-term successful language use? From a strictly linguistic point of view, we have to adopt an Orwellian principle, that all structures are equal . . . The remedial instinct advises us to teach them all—but we know we cannot teach them all. So which ones do we retain, and which do we give up? I would hazard a guess about the pervasiveness, and thus the fundamental value of *certain* clause structures, for instance, but not all of them (might not P be able to survive without ever knowing, say, the Subject-Verb-Object-Complement construction, as in *I called John a fool?*). But is it even meaningful to ask, in effect, the question 'Are some structures more equal than others?'—such questions as: is *will* more useful than *can*? Are pronouns more useful than determiners? Are irregular verbs Type A more useful than Type B? Or, to consider an example in more detail: which prepositions to work on? There are about 150 prepositions in English. I list them in Table 6, but do not include the many 'complex' prepositions of the type *in front of* or *in accordance with*. No teaching programme has yet been constructed which deals with all of them, so how does one decide which to choose? Language acquisition information could help, but so far only a handful of prepositions have been studied as a part of early learning; frequency information could also help, but no reliable word counts for spoken language exist (it would be unwise to generalize from those based on written samples, such as Thorndike & Lorge 1944). Some prepositions are so specialized or formal that few Ts would grieve over their absence—and doubtless there are large numbers of people who have lived perfectly happy and successful lives without ever using such words as *notwithstanding* or *circa*. But how to evaluate the 100 or so that are neither the first nor the last to be acquired? And how to evaluate the larger question: whether to spend a large amount of time on preposition training is in itself justifiable, given the competing claims of auxiliary verbs, determiners, conjunctions, and much more?

These questions are relevant for all levels of clinical linguistic enquiry, not just for grammar. They can be asked, in exactly the same way, concerning phonology. There are over 300 consonants,

Table 6   Single-word and some two-word prepositions

Monosyllabic	Polysyllabic	Marginal	Two-word
as	about	bar	as for
at	above	barring	but for
but	across	concerning	except for
by	after	considering	
down	against	excepting	apart from
for	along	excluding	as from
from	amid(st)	failing	aside from
in	among(st)	following	away from
like	anti	given	
near	around	granted	ahead of
of	atop	including	as of
off	before	less	back of
on	behind	minus	because of
out	below	pending	devoid of
past	beneath	plus	exclusive of
per	beside	regarding	inside of
pro	besides	respecting	instead of
re	between	save	irrespective of
round	beyond	times	off of
sans	circa	touching	out of
since	despite	wanting	outside of
than	during		regardless of
through	except		upwards of
till	inside		void of
to	into		
up	notwithstanding		according to
vs	onto		as to
via	opposite		close to
with	outside		contrary to
	over		due to
	pace		near to
	pending		next to
	throughout		on to
	toward(s)		owing to
	under		preliminary to
	underneath		preparatory to
	unlike		previous to
	until		prior to
	upon		pursuant to
	versus		subsequent to
	vis-a-vis		thanks to
	within		etc.
	without		

vowels and consonant clusters distributed over initial, medial and final positions in words in English. The criteria of language acquisition and frequency of use, along with a few other criteria usually discussed in the context of phonology (such as functional load and phonetic salience), will help to suggest some useful foci for early learning and some advanced patterns which one might be happy to ignore (such as final -CCCC clusters, as in *glimpsed* or *twelfths*). But in between . . . ? How should we decide which phonological contrasts are worth concentrating upon more than others? And what about the higher-order question of whether it is worth spending proportionately more time on phonology than grammar?

Lastly, the same questions force themselves on us again, in relation to the lexicon—only here, they come in their thousands. At least in phonology, we are dealing with a mere few hundred categories of sound, and in grammar perhaps with as many as a thousand constructions; but in vocabulary, we are dealing with a long-term goal of tens of thousands of items. The same general considerations of acquisition and frequency apply in theory, but in practice the literature has little to offer, in the absence of much empirical research into the frequency and learning of spoken vocabulary. The graded lists devised for the teaching of reading are sometimes used as a way into the problem, but this is not to be recommended, partly in view of the arbitrary way in which all such lists have been devised, and partly because there is no clear correspondence between spoken and reading vocabulary anyway (as we know, intuitively, as adults, with our passive reading vocabulary being far in excess of our active speaking vocabulary).

To summarize. Even if personnel and resources were inexhaustible, the nature of language handicap makes it impossible to teach the whole of the language in a systematic or successful way. Ts therefore have to be selective in what they teach. This selectivity has to be carried out on a principled basis, if a coherent and consistent remedial practice is to develop among all who are involved with P. The principles have to relate to both the structural and functional dimensions of language, if a balanced linguistic ability is to emerge. But given the limited progress which has been made in the statistical and acquisitional study of language, under either of these headings, it is impossible to see how any such principles can be operationalized. The conclusion is plain: it is not possible to arrive at a coherent remedial linguistic philosophy, at the present time.

If this reasoning is correct, there are only a limited number of positions which students of language handicap can adopt. The first is to become a student of something else, such as bricklaying (for which we probably have excellent qualifications). The second is to reject the principle of remedial efficacy as a primary goal, and concentrate on some kind of compensatory programme. The third is to retain the remedial goal, but to rationalize the selectivity principles on which we work, in relation to the short- and long-term demands imposed on P. I would very much like to see a proper discussion of the factors which would enable us to choose between the second and third of these alternatives. I cannot present a balanced account myself, because I have never been involved in compensatory programmes. But I can, at least, sketch out the implications of the third position, as far as research priorities in clinical linguistics are concerned. It would seem that, in order to operationalize the selectivity principle, we need at least three kinds of information. First, we need to know the absolute limits of the language learning that the nature of P's handicap imposes upon him. This means a programme of follow-up studies on a large scale, focusing on the older age-range of children, in the first instance. Until we know what these limits are, a principled discussion of selectivity cannot begin. If we know that structure X is *never* satisfactorily acquired, using present-day intervention techniques, then and only then are we in a position to discuss whether it is worthwhile trying to teach it, using different techniques, or to drop it altogether from the curriculum. Alternatively, if we know that it is clearly acquired, or partly acquired, this knowledge will condition our views about the amount and kind of attention we pay to it. In short, because knowledge of the end-point of development is a *sine qua non* of progress, at least a third of our research efforts ought to be devoted to this goal. At present, the figure must be point nought nought something.

Secondly, we need to work towards a functional model which will enable us to evaluate the structural and pragmatic properties of language in longitudinal terms. The model would do more than has often been suggested in proposals to 'quantify' intervention. It would not only provide an estimate of the amount of time needed to establish a property in P, and of the point in development at which this time would be best spent; it would also assign a weighting to a property, which would indicate the short- or long-term usefulness of teaching it to P. For example, the use of the comparative construction would probably achieve a high weighting, because of its known importance in relation to the development of certain cognitive skills in young children, as well as its specific role in such areas as the teaching of mathematics. By contrast, the use of cleft sentence constructions would probably carry a fairly low weighting, as their linguistic role seems to be much more subtle and stylistically 'optional'. Plainly, the two research areas most involved in this work would be psycholinguistics (language acquisition, in particular) and sociolinguistics (variety analysis, in particular). Both areas would need to be serviced by descriptive and theoretical linguistics—the former, because it is necessary to arrive at statistical norms for the use of the various properties of language; the latter, because the more we know about language universals, and the constraints which affect them, the more motivation we will have for an analogous theory of linguistic breakdown (cf. p.86). The whole research package should take up most of the second third of our research effort.

And the third third? We carry on as before—transcribing, describing, analysing, hypothesizing, trying out remedial procedures—but hopefully, now, always looking ahead, to the linguistic demands of the school syllabus, and of P's social world, no longer satisfied with teaching 'X', but aiming to know that it is 'useful X': not just 'verbs', but 'useful verbs'; not just 'fricatives', but 'useful fricatives in useful positions'; and so on (cf. Chapter 4). Everyone hopes and believes that their remedial teaching falls within this utilitarian perspective; but the spontaneous carry-over from T's clinic to P's world, which would be the evidence of this achievement, is a rare event indeed. Perhaps the most ambitious of all the aims of clinical linguistics (in the broadest sense, to include clinical psycho- and socio-linguistics) is to replace 'hope and believe' by 'know', in the last sentence, and thus to be able to guarantee the smoothest possible transition between the restricted, structure-orientated world of remedial language teaching and the creative, open-ended world of employment, leisure, imagination and the spirit. Ambitious this goal may be; yet progress towards its achievement is crucial, for without it, the scientific element in the training of the remedial language professional cannot be justified, nor the need for professional intervention defended.

References

Albert, M.L., Goodglass, H., Helm, N.A., Rubens, A.B. and Alexander, M.P. 1981. *Clinical Aspects of Dysphasia*. Vienna: Springer.

Aram, D.M. and Nation, J.E. 1980. Preschool language disorders and subsequent language and academic difficulties. *Journal of Communication Disorders* 13, pp.159-70.

Aram, D.M. and Nation, J.E. 1982. *Child Language Disorders*. St. Louis: Mosby.

Argyle, M. 1967. *The Psychology of Interpersonal Behaviour*. Harmondsworth: Penguin.

Baldie, B.J. 1976. The acquisition of the passive voice. *Journal of Child Language* 3, pp.331-48.

Berry, M.F. and Eisenson, J. 1956. *Speech Disorders*. London: Peter Owen.

Bullock Report. 1975. *A Language for Life*. London: H.M.S.O.

Byers Brown, B. 1981. *Speech Therapy: Principles and Practice*. Edinburgh: Churchill Livingstone.

Byrne, B. 1981. Deficient syntactic control in poor readers: is a weak phonetic memory code responsible? *AppliedPsycholinguistics* 2, pp.201-12.

Chazan, M., ed. 1973. *Compensatory Education*. London: Butterworths.

Clark, H.H. and Clark, E.V. 1977. *Psychology and Language: an Introduction to Psycholinguistics*. New York: Harcourt, Brace and Jovanovich.

Cocking, R. and McHale, S. 1981. A comparative study of the use of pictures and objects in assessing children's receptive and productive language. *Journal of Child Language* 8, pp.1-13.

Code, C. and Muller, D.J., eds. 1983. *Aphasia Therapy*. London: Edward Arnold.

Cole, M. 1967. *Fogie: the Life of Elsie Fogerty*. London: Peter Davies.

Coltheart, M. 1980. Deep dyslexia: a review of the syndrome. In Coltheart *et al.*, *Deep Dyslexia*, pp.22-47.

—— 1983. Aphasia therapy research: a single-case study approach. In Code and Muller, eds., *Aphasia Therapy*, pp.193-302.

Coltheart, M., Patterson, K. and Marshall, J.C., eds. 1980. *Deep Dyslexia*. London: Routledge and Kegan Paul.

Critchley, M. 1970. *Aphasiology*. London: Edward Arnold.

Crystal, D. 1969. *Prosodic Systems and Intonation in English*. Cambridge: Cambridge University Press.

—— 1971. *Linguistics*. Harmondsworth: Penguin.

—— 1972. The case of linguistics: a prognosis. *British Journal of Disorders of Communication* 7, pp.3-16.

—— 1976. *Child Language, Learning and Linguistics*. London: Edward Arnold.

—— 1979. Reading, grammar and the line. In D. Thackray, ed., *Growth in Reading*. London: Ward Lock Education.

—— 1981. *Clinical Linguistics*. Vienna: Springer.

—— 1982a. *Profiling Linguistic Disability*. London: Edward Arnold.

—— 1982b. Pseudo-controversy in linguistic theory. In D. Crystal, ed., *Linguistic Controversies*. London: Edward Arnold, pp. 16-24.

—— forthcoming. Language input variables in aphasia. Paper given at the Symposium in Advances in Aphasiology, Medical Society of London, 1983. To appear in *Progress in Aphasiology*. New York: Raven Press.

Crystal, D. and Davy, D. 1969. *Investigating English Style*. London: Longman.

—— 1975. *Advanced Conversational English*. London: Longman.

Crystal, D., Fletcher, P. & Garman, M. 1976. *The Grammatical Analysis of Language Disability*. London: Edward Arnold.

De Ajuriaguerra, J., Jaeggi, A., Guignard, F., Kocker, F., Maquard, M., Roth, S. and Schmid, E. 1976. The development and prognosis of dysphasia in children. In D.M. Morehead and A.E. Morehead, eds., *Normal and Deficient Child Language*. Baltimore: University Park Press, pp.345-85.

De Vito, J.A. 1971.*Psycholinguistics*. Indianapolis: Bobbs-Merrill.

Doughty, P., Pearce, J. and Thornton, G. 1971. *Language in Use*. London: Edward Arnold.

Edwards, M.L. 1974. Perception and production in child phonology: the testing of four hypotheses. *Journal of Child Language* 1, pp.205-19.

Edwards, R.P.A. and Gibbon, V. 1964. *Words Your Children Use*.

London: Burke.

Eisenson, J. 1973. *Adult Aphasia: Assessment and Treatment*. Englewood Cliffs, NJ: Prentice-Hall.

Emerick, L. and Hatten, J.T. 1974. *Diagnosis and Evaluation in Speech Pathology*. Englewood Cliffs, NJ: Prentice-Hall.

Ervin-Tripp, S. and Slobin, S.I. 1966. Psycholinguistics. *Annual Review of Psychology* 17, pp.435-74.

Firth, J.R. 1948. Sounds and prosodies. *Transactions of the Philological Society*, pp.127-52.

Fletcher, P. 1985. *The Child's Learning of English*. Oxford: Blackwell.

Furrow, D., Nelson, K. and Benedict, H. 1979. Mothers' speech to children and syntactic development: some simple relationships. *Journal of Child Language* 6, pp.423-42.

Gallagher, T.M. and Prutting, C.A., eds. 1983. *Pragmatic Assessment and Intervention Issues in Language*. San Diego: College-Hill.

Garvey, M. and Gordon, N. 1973. A follow-up study of children with disorders of speech development. *British Journal of Disorders of Communication* 8, pp.17-28.

Gearhart, B.R. 1981. *Learning Disabilities: Educational Strategies*. Third edition. St. Louis: Mosby.

Gleitman, L.R., Newport, E.L. and Gleitman, H. 1984. The current status of the motherese hypothesis. *Journal of Child Language* 11, pp.43-79.

Goodglass, H. 1968. Studies on the grammar of aphasics. In S. Rosenberg and J.H. Koplin, eds., *Developments in Applied Psycholinguistics Research*. New York: Macmillan, pp.177-208.

—— 1976. Agrammatism. In H. Whitaker and H.A. Whitaker, eds., *Studies in Neurolinguistics*, I. London: Academic Press, pp. 237-60.

Goodglass, H. and Kaplan, E. 1972. *The Assessment of Aphasia and Related Disorders*. Philadelphia: Lea and Febiger.

Greene, J. 1972. *Psycholinguistics: Chomsky and Psychology*. Harmondsworth: Penguin.

Griffiths, C.P.S. 1969. A follow-up study of children with disorders of speech. *British Journal of Disorders of Communication* 4, pp. 46-56.

Grunwell, P. 1981. *The Nature of Phonological Disability in Children*. London: Academic Press.

Grunwell, P., *et al.* 1980. Progress report: the phonetic representation of disordered speech. *British Journal of Disorders of Communication* 15, pp.215-20.

Gumperz, J.J. and Hymes, D. 1972. *Directions in Sociolinguistics: the Ethnography of Communication*. New York: Holt, Rinehart and Winston.

Hall, P.K. and Tomblin, J.B. 1978. A follow-up study of children with articulation and language disorders. *Journal of Speech and Hearing Disorders* 43, pp.227-41.

Hall Powers, M. 1963. Functional disorders of articulation—symptomatology and aetiology. In L.E. Travis, ed., *Handbook of Speech Pathology*, pp.707-69.

Halliday, M.A.K. 1961. Categories of the theory of grammar. *Word*, 17, pp.241-92.

Hockett, C.F. 1958. *A Course in Modern Linguistics*. New York: Macmillan.

Hockett, C.F. and Altmann, S. 1968. A note on design features. In T.A. Sebeok, ed., *Animal Communication: Techniques of Study and Results of Research*. Bloomington: Indiana University Press, pp. 61-72.

Hörmann, H. 1979. *Psycholinguistics: an Introduction to Research and Theory*. (Trans. H.H.Stern and P.Leppman.) Second edition. New York: Springer.

Hutt, E. 1973. *Language Therapy*, Vol.2. London: Invalid Children's Aid Association.

Ingram, D. 1976. *Phonological Disability in Children*. London: Edward Arnold.

Ingram, T.T.S., Mason, A.W. and Blackburn, I. 1970. A retrospective study of 82 children with reading disability. *Developmental Medicine and Child Neurology* 12, pp.271-81.

Jakobson, R. 1954. Two aspects of language and two types of aphasic disturbances. Reprinted in *Selected Writings*, Vol.2, 1971. The Hague: Mouton, pp.239-59.

—— 1971. Linguistic types of aphasia. In *Selected Writings*, Vol.2. The Hague: Mouton, pp.307-33.

—— 1980. On aphasic disorders from a linguistic angle. In R.Jakobson, *The Framework of Language*. Ann Arbor: Michigan Studies in the Humanities, pp.93-111.

Johnson, K. and Porter, D. 1983. *Perspectives in Communicative Language Teaching*. London: Academic Press.

Krommer-Benz, M. 1977. *World Guide to Terminological Activities*. Munich.

Lee, L. 1966. Developmental sentence types. *Journal of Speech and Hearing Disorders* 31, pp.311-30.

Leech, G.N. 1983. *Principles of Pragmatics*. London: Longman.

Lesser, R. 1978. *Linguistic Investigations of Aphasia*. London: Edward Arnold.

Levinson, S. 1983. *Pragmatics*. Cambridge: Cambridge University Press.

Limber, J. 1973. The genesis of complex sentences. In T.E. Moore, ed., *Cognitive Development and the Acquisition of Language*. New York: Academic Press, pp.169-85.

Lingua. 1967. *Word Classes*. Amsterdam: North-Holland.

Ludlow, C.L. 1981. Recovery and rehabilitation of adult aphasic patients: relevant research advances. In R.W. Rieber, ed., *Communication Disorders*. New York: Plenum Press, pp.149-77.

Lyle, J.G. 1970. Certain antenatal, perinatal and developmental variables and reading retardation in middle class boys. *Child Development* 41, pp.481-91.

Lyons, J. 1977. *Semantics*. Cambridge: Cambridge University Press.

Mackay, D., Thompson, B. and Schaub, I. 1970. *Breakthrough to Literacy*. London: Longman.

McTear, M. 1985. *The Development of Conversational Ability in Children*. Oxford: Blackwell.

Maratsos, M. 1976. *The Use of Definite and Indefinite Reference in Young Children*. Cambridge: Cambridge University Press.

Marsh, G., Gearhart, C. and Gearhart, B. 1978. *The Learning Disabled Adolescent: Program Alternatives in the Secondary School*. St.Louis: Mosby.

Martin, D. 1974. Some objections to the term 'apraxia of speech'. *Journal of Speech and Hearing Disorders* 39, pp.53-64.

Milisen, R. 1966. Articulatory problems—organic conditions and the disorder of articulation. In R. Rieber and R. Brubaker, eds., *Speech Pathology: an International Study of the Science*. Amsterdam: North Holland, pp.301-20.

Miller, J., Yoder, D.E. and Schiefelbusch, R. 1983. *Contemporary Issues in Language Intervention*. Rockville, Md.: American Speech—Language—Hearing Association.

Moon, C. 1979. Categorization of miscues arising from textual weakness. In D. Thackray, ed., *Growth in Reading*. London: Ward Lock Education, pp.135-46.

—— 1981. Identification of readability factors. In J. Chapman, ed., *The Reader and the Text*. London: Ward Lock Education.

Morley, M. 1972. *The Development and Disorders of Speech in Childhood*. Third edition. Edinburgh: Churchill Livingstone.

Morley, M. and Fox, J. 1969. Disorders of articulation: theory and therapy. *British Journal of Disorders of Communication* 4, pp. 151-65.

Morton, J. 1980. Two auditory parallels to deep dyslexia. In Coltheart *et al.*, *Deep Dyslexia*, pp.189-96.

National Advisory Committee on Handicapped Children. 1968. Special Education for Handicapped Children. First Annual Report. Washington, Office of Education: Department of Health, Education and Welfare.

Nicolosi, L., Harryman, E. and Kresheck, J. 1978. *Terminology of Communication Disorders: Speech, Language, Hearing*. Baltimore: Williams and Wilkins.

Ochs, E. and Schieffelin, B. 1979. *Developmental Pragmatics*. New York: Academic Press.

Osgood, C.E. and Sebeok, T.A. 1954. *Psycholinguistics: a Survey of Theory and Research Problems*. Supplement to *Journal of Abnormal and Social Psychology* 49.

Perera, K. 1982. The assessment of linguistic difficulty in reading material. In R. Carter, ed., *Linguistics and the Teacher*. London: Routledge and Kegan Paul, pp.101-13.

Perello, J. 1977. *Lexicon de Communicologia*. Barcelona: Ed.Augusta.

Quirk, R., Greenbaum, S., Leech, G.N. and Svartvik, J. forthcoming. *A Grammar of English*. London: Longman.

Quirk, R. and Svartvik, J. 1966. *Investigating Linguistic Acceptability*. The Hague: Mouton.

Quirk Report. 1972. *Speech Therapy Services*. London: H.M.S.O.

Raban, B. 1981. *Line Breaks in Texts for Young Children*. SSRC Report HR 6390/1. London: Social Science Research Council.

—— 1982. *Vocabulary of 5-year-olds*. University of Reading.

Robbins, S.D. 1951. *A Dictionary of Speech Pathology and Therapy*. Cambridge, Mass.: Sci-Art Publications.

Saffran, E.M., Bogyo, L.C., Schwartz, M.F. and Marin, O.S.M. 1980. Does deep dyslexia reflect right-hemisphere reading? In Coltheart *et al.*, *Deep Dyslexia*, pp.381-406.

Sager, J.C. and Johnson, R.L. 1978. Terminology: the state of the art. *AILA Bulletin* 1 (22), 1-12.

Sarno, M.T. 1969. *The Functional Communication Profile*. New York: Institute of Rehabilitation Medicine.

Sebeok, T.A., Hayes, A.S. and Bateson, M.C., eds., 1964. *Approaches to Semiotics*. The Hague: Mouton.

Skinner, C.M., Wirz, S.L. and Thompson, I.M. 1983. The Edinburgh functional communication profile—an interim report. *Bulletin of the College of Speech Therapists* 371, pp.1-3.

Slobin, D.I. 1971. *Psycholinguistics*. Glenview, Ill.: Scott, Foresman.

Steinberg, D.D. 1982. *Psycholinguistics: Language, Mind and World*.

London: Longman.

Tarnopol, L. and Tarnopol, M., eds. 1976. *Reading Disabilities: an International Perspective.* Baltimore: University Park Press.

Thorndike, E.L. and Lorge, I. 1944. *The Teacher's Word Book of 30,000 Words.* New York: Columbia University.

Travis, L.E. ed. 1963. *Handbook of Speech Pathology.* Second edition. New York: Appleton-Century-Crofts.

Tymchuk, A.J. 1973. *The Mental Retardation Dictionary.* Los Angeles: Western Psychological Services.

Van Riper, C. and Irwin, J.V. 1958. *Voice and Articulation.* Second edition. London: Pitman Medical.

Vellutino, F.R. 1979. *Dyslexia: Theory and Research.* Cambridge, Mass.: M.I.T. Press.

Weiner, P.S. 1974. A language-delayed child at adolescence. *Journal of Speech and Hearing Disorders* 39, pp.202-12.

Wells, G., ed. 1980. *Learning through Interaction.* Cambridge: Cambridge University Press.

Whurr, R. 1982. Towards a typology of aphasic impairment. In Crystal, ed., *Linguistic Controversies*, pp.239-57.

Wolpaw, T., Nation, J.E. and Aram, D.M. 1977. Developmental language disorders: a follow-up study. *Selected Papers in Language and Phonology*, Vol.1. Evanston, Ill.: Institute for Continuing Professional Education.

World Health Organization. 1974. *Glossary of Mental Disorders and Guide to their Classification.* Geneva.

Wren, C.T., ed. 1983. *Language Learning Disabilities.* Rockville, Md.: Aspen.

Index

DATE DUE

MR 1 3 '89			